"Reading this book is like having a ch ...... .e and supportive. Lauren's Change4Good prog ...... It follows 10 essential, yet basic common-sense p, ... practical and easy to learn. What I really respect is that not o ...... Lauren provide an understandable, holistic approach to nutrition but her emphasis on being mindful of who you are, discovering your motivations, and taking a personal inventory on where you are in life. Then, you have a choice: do you truly want to change or not? She is a living example of her program. As a physician, I admire Lauren's Change4Good program, and am delighted that she has written a sound and realistic step-by-step guide for you. I hope you enjoy the program as much as I am."
Dr. Ivy Cheng, MD, FRCP, FACEM, dABEM, Dip of SM, DiMM
Emergency Physician and Sports Medicine Physician

"Finally, a book that maps out how each and every one of us can Change (our long-time unhealthy eating/exercising patterns) 4Good. This book is beautifully written, impressively practical and hits on all the key points that easily guide us toward lasting life-style change. This book is a gift to all of us who have struggled navigating our way through yo-yo diets and unrealistic exercise programs, only to find ourselves back where we started or worse! Change4Good shines a light on the heart of the matter and helps us to rebuild from a fresh and healthy foundation. It is rich in content, foundationally solid and most importantly, it is built around 10 realistic principles that will guide you toward permanent change. "
Lorraine Gilks, B.Ed., CPCC, ACC, CH, NLP
Professor, Workplace Wellness & Health Promotion Graduate Program, Centennial College
Managing Partner, 3P Coaching

"I have genuine respect for Lauren Jawno's knowledge and many years of experience. In Change4Good Lauren has put together information that is simple, easy to implement and flexible. The extent of information is powerful yet easy to understand and relate to with the use of practical examples. If you are ready to get real about your health and life balance then you have found the ultimate solution in Change4Good by Lauren Jawno!"
Vera Bond, BA in Kinesiology, ACE, NASM
Founder and Director of Inspired Energy International
Former Reebok Master Trainer

"This is quite simply the best book about food and nutrition that I've read. It takes you out of the mindset of quick fixes or denying yourself pleasure and puts you on track to understanding your relationship with food, grasping the concepts you need to make good food choices and live a healthier, happier life. Finally there's someone who gets it."
From the Foreward by Mark Sutcliffe
Founder of iRun Magazine and the Author of Why I Run: The Remarkable Journey of the Ordinary Runner

"To stay competitive over my 25 year career as one of Canada's top track and field athletes, I have worked with many experts in sports nutrition and physiology. Lauren's Change4Good principles have given me additional tools to not only keep my eating on track in my busy life as an athlete, a professional and a mother but to also help me identify where I can make changes to optimize my performance and success."

Tania Jones
Canadian Marathon Champion, National Team Member, Top ranked Masters Runner

"Lauren has told her authentic story, sharing her educational expertise and personal experiences to provide a practical fitness, nutrition, and 'way of thinking' road map for those who want to live a healthy, balanced life. Her 10 core principles are easy strategies that can help anyone avoid the pitfalls and overcome the barriers that so often disrupt the essential habits required for living well. Based on changes in attitude, behaviour and lifestyle, Lauren's Change4Good program offers simple and flexible advice for anyone looking to control their weight and achieve long lasting success."

Dr. Scott D. Howitt, BA, MSC, DC, FRCCSS(C), FCCRS(C)
Sports and Rehabilitation Specialist Chiropractor, Acupuncture
Director of Sports Performance Centres Ltd.

Lauren Jawno has been my personal trainer for the past seven years, and has trained my husband and two sons as well. In addition to training, she provides nutritional advice when needed and has also helped us through various running and other sports injuries. Her book is full of great advice for those not fortunate enough to have her as a trainer.

Karen Boehlert
Client

"Change4Good is so simple - anyone can do this! Lauren has put together everything you need to succeed in a well written, well organized tool. Forget the gimmicks, the expensive diets and so-called miraculous weight loss drugs - they don't work. I've tried many of them too. Change4Good works because it's flexible and you can tailor it to your preferences. I've trained with Lauren for several years - applying these principles in my life has helped me manage a rigorous schedule, career transitions and bounce back quickly from two difficult pregnancies. Change4Good will help you get healthy and stay healthy."

Dr. Leah Watson, MD, FRCPC
Emergency Physician
University Health Network and Sunnybrook Health Sciences Centre

CHANGE4GOOD

The Ten Essentials for Food, Fitness and the Good Life

BY

LAUREN JAWNO

WITH

FRAN SCHUMER

authorHOUSE®

AuthorHouse™
1663 Liberty Drive
Bloomington, IN 47403
www.authorhouse.com
Phone: 1-800-839-8640

First published by AuthorHouse   01/2012

ISBN: 978-1-4678-7693-3 (sc)
ISBN: 978-1-4678-7692-6 (hc)
ISBN: 978-1-4678-7691-9 (ebk)

Library of Congress Control Number: 2011961503

Printed in the United States of America

DISCLAIMER AND NOTICES

The content of this book is intended for information purposes only and should not be used in any way to diagnose, prevent or treat any illness; or used as a substitute for personalized medical advice.

The primary objective of this book is to present and highlight lifestyle, fitness and nutritionally significant information, to offer guidelines and recommendations for improving and maintaining the general state of the reader's health, wellness and nutritional intake.

The author shall not be held responsible for the information or any inadvertent errors or omissions of the information or if the information presented herein fails to deliver results expected by the reader.

The products and nutritional supplements outlined in this book are not endorsed by the author nor does the author receive any compensation for their mention.

DEDICATION

In loving memory of my mother, Esther Cecile Jawno; not by words alone but in her life, she taught me about integrity, courage, grace and selflessness. She taught me how to look up and not to give up. Her spirit informs every page of this book.

In gratitude to my brother, Jonathan, his work ethic has been my role model; his kindness and generosity, my fuel. Nothing I have accomplished would be possible without him. I love and respect him more than words can express.

ACKNOWLEDGEMENTS

It is with enormous humility, gratitude and appreciation that I would like to thank the following people for their support, guidance and assistance in helping me complete this book.

Firstly, to my core team who have been instrumental in making this dream a reality. To Fran Schumer, who saw the value in my work; my gratitude to her for her persistence, inquiring mind and most of all for helping to make my voice heard through this work. Jackie Mungal, my *artiste* extraordinaire, who manifested endless patience and creativity in designing and editing this book. Jackie, thank you for your time, valuable advice, unconditional support and friendship. To Larry Grabb and his amazing team at AuthorHouse™ who have graced me with their guidance, insight and assistance.

Throughout my career, my clients have honoured me with their trust and loyalty; their unflagging interest and enthusiasm has and continues to sustain me. My many colleagues and teachers; and the select group of mentors I have been fortunate enough to encounter throughout my career have inspired and encouraged me, always challenging me to do my best and be my best, in all of my endeavours. Thanks to you for your support.

My sincere gratitude to the small group of people who took valuable time out of their busy schedules to read through drafts of this book and provide me with constructive and crucial feedback. A special thanks to Mark Sutcliffe for his unfaltering support of my work and this book. I am privileged to write for his magazine, iRun, and am incredibly honoured to have had him write the forward to my book.

Thank you to Tailor Medical, for generously allowing me to use the clinic to film the fitness videos for my website, to Priscilla for graciously agreeing to be my fitness model, Claudia for doing our make-up and Ryan for your creative vision and professionalism.

My ex-husband, Wayne, with whom I shared a huge part of my life, was integral in supporting the growth of my career throughout our marriage. I cherish the happy times we shared and will always remain grateful.

To my extended family, but especially Colin and Brenda, Stacey, Gillian and Joe, and Bonnie and Mel; you all provide a loving voice of reason that helps keep me on track and for which I am always thankful.

To my inner circle of exceptional friends – what would I do without all of you and the wonderful friendships we share? Priscilla you help keep me grounded and motivated in so many ways. Claudia, you are without a doubt not only the best road trip buddy anyone could wish for but also a loyal confidant. Salim, your down-to-earth and sincere friendship is a breath of fresh air that I appreciate every day. Michelle, even though you are a world away, I know you are always there for me, wishing me only the best of everything. Loren your loyalty and friendship has stood the test of time and for that I am so grateful. Nicky you lovingly tolerate me on my very worst days and at the same time have the incredible ability to make me laugh like no-one else. Ilana, my very dear friend - you are always there for me, no matter what - my life would not be complete without you in it. Thanks to all of you for your genuine interest, love and endless encouragement.

Finally and most importantly, to my loving family, who, although at opposite ends of the world, living on three different continents and spanning a multitude of time zones; all in their own unique way never stop supporting me, believing in me and encouraging me to be the best I can be in everything I do every day of my life. To David, Dianne, Kerri and Jareth in Australia, who love and care for me in every possible way. To Jonathan, Natanya, Shai, Atara, Nina and Nurit in South Africa, for the incredible love, kindness and support you bring into my life every single day even though you, too, are worlds away. And to my loving father, who teaches me all the right things: honesty, integrity and the importance of believing in and living up to one's potential. Thanks to you, Dad. Thanks to all.

Table of Contents

Table of Contents

Foreword

I've never fully understood the strange relationship we have with food. Most of us don't know very much about food, and what we do know is more likely to be culinary than nutritional – how to prepare it rather than how to get the most out of what's inside it. We don't learn much about nutrition in school, aren't inclined to explore it more as adults and we typically make choices – healthy and unhealthy – based on taste rather than nourishment.

There is something deeply personal and psychological about food; it's connected to our environment, our self-esteem, and our relationships with other people. Food is fundamental to our existence and yet we know so little about how to benefit from it to make our lives better and longer. I'm typical of this. Because I run a lot, my weight is under control. But that doesn't mean I don't have food issues. I have a massive sweet tooth so I eat a lot of desserts. And food is deeply connected to my psyche; I eat to reward myself for accomplishment and to compensate for disappointment.

I generally eat healthy and do my best to get the prescribed servings of fruits and vegetables, but I can also eat a row of cookies in three minutes or less. If there's a bowl of potato chips in the room, I'm constantly aware of it until it's consumed; not able to devote my complete attention to anything else.

I try to learn more about food but most of the information that's available isn't very useful. Cookbooks and cooking shows are all about taste – just look at the butter in some of those recipes.

The diet industry certainly doesn't help us with our lack of knowledge about food. Indeed, if anything, it capitalizes on our ignorance rather than helps us overcome it.

Once every few years, a new method of dieting is introduced that becomes the latest craze. It makes someone a lot of money but it doesn't really solve the problem. If any of these diets worked, would obesity rates be increasing?

These fad diets are the get-rich-quick schemes of personal health. They promise the impossible but as long as you put your money in, it doesn't really matter to the proponents whether they deliver the results you wanted. You may get short-term results, but as soon as you go back to your old habits, you'll start gaining again.

Even the more substantial weight-loss programs offer mostly fleeting success; many of them address only the scientific and not the emotional and psychological aspects of food. Eat less and you'll lose weight. Cutting calories sounds good on paper, but when you're sitting in front of the TV and you've got the munchies, you have a choice between denying yourself pleasure or violating your program. Either way, you lose.

Most of these programs are trying to fix a problem rather than replace a lifestyle. They propose rigid rules that may work for a few weeks or months, but ultimately are unsustainable. They focus almost exclusively on what you should and shouldn't eat, and devote little attention to the factors that are causing you to have an unhealthy relationship with food.

And yet so many people are drawn to these flawed solutions. They think there's a quick solution to a problem that is usually a lifetime in the making. They think that overnight; they can fix their deeply engrained, long-standing habits around food or trick themselves into behaving differently or their bodies into shedding pounds.

Nobody would train for a marathon or try to pass a law exam using an easy scheme or trick. There are fundamental principles at play that most people respect when it comes to most things that are difficult and life-changing. But adjust your approach to eating, your entire mentality about food? For some reason, the prevailing mentality is that losing pounds has nothing to do with principles and everything to do with tricks and gimmicks.

Finally, though, there's someone who gets it. In this book, Lauren Jawno demonstrates that eating healthy isn't about giving up anything. It's about adopting a better lifestyle and all the benefits that go with it. It's not about a constant battle or living in denial. It's about principles that will allow you to live completely.

Lauren has been a regular contributor to iRun magazine and a recurring guest on our radio show and podcast and the feedback to her expertise has always been extremely positive. And she hasn't just worked with clients to help them achieve a better lifestyle, she's overcome her own struggles with food and weight gain that she documents here in refreshingly candid detail.

This is quite simply the best book about food and nutrition that I've read. It takes you out of the mindset of quick fixes or denying yourself pleasure and puts you on track to understanding your relationship with food, grasping the concepts you need to make good food choices and living a healthier, happier life.

Mark Sutcliffe is the founder of iRun magazine and he author of *Why I Run: The Remarkable Journey of the Ordinary Runner*
Ottawa, Canada
October 2011

My Story

The first client I ever diagnosed was myself; I was six years old and came home from my first day of Grade 1 convinced that I was fat. The funny thing was, I wasn't. What shocks me now is that even as a first-grader, I was self-conscious of my weight. Unbeknownst to me then, my weight would become an issue that would consume me for decades. But it would also ultimately be the catalyst to incredible self-growth and understanding.

Grade 1 was significant in another way. I started to play tennis. Within a few years it became a defining part of my life as I began to play more seriously. The warm, sunny days in South Africa, where I was raised, were conducive to long afternoons and evenings on the courts.

Tennis wasn't just my hobby; it was my life. I approached my tennis and training as if I were a nationally ranked player. Most weekends and every day after school, I'd change into my tennis clothes and spend the rest of the day training, both on and off the court. I always played for the top-ranked teams at each of my schools, and accumulated a collection of trophies over the years. Tennis instilled in me the value of hard work; it taught me discipline and sportsmanship. To this day, the skills I learned on the courts benefit me off the courts as well. As much as I loved tennis, and still do, I realized years later that there was much more to my drive and dedication than the mere passion for the game.

By the end of grade eleven in high school, I'd reached my full adult height of 5'6" and I weighed a reasonable 130 pounds. This brief period, in which I hardly thought about weight or dieting, ended rather abruptly with the beginning of grade twelve. In order to gain entrance to the university I wanted to attend, I needed to immerse myself in study. Overnight, I transformed myself from athlete to scholar. Sitting at my desk, I gained 30 pounds.

Enter Lauren Jawno, the chronic dieter. I grew frantic at the amount of weight I had gained. At 165 pounds, I was certain that I'd be the fattest freshman at the University of Cape Town. I longed for some pill that would obliterate the problem. My wish was granted initially in the form of a prescription for laxatives and later, appetite suppressants, both handed to me by my family doctor. In no time, I was hooked. I did not have much of an appetite and I took so many laxatives that I had to run to different pharmacies in order to avoid arousing suspicion. "You were just here," the pharmacist would say when I showed up within days of having picked up my last prescription. "Oh, I lost it," I'd lie.

Three months into my first term at college, I lost 30 and then 40 pounds. I ate little and I practically lived in the bathroom. I viewed weight as my problem, but in retrospect, there were other issues. For one, I was living away from home for the first time, and lonely. For another, the absence of competitive sports in my life had left a void. If I was no longer Lauren the tennis player, then who was I? In search of some other identity, I focused on my appearance – which to me, of course, meant my weight. But weight wasn't the real problem, neither was my loneliness or the absence of competitive tennis in my life.

As a result during the next twelve years, I gained and lost the same 30-40 pounds dozens of times, and on all kinds of diets: Weight Watchers®, the Zone Diet®, South Beach Diet®, the Cabbage Soup Diet®, the Master Cleanse© and some of my own devising (ketchup and green peas; rice and water). No matter how wacky a regimen my clients present me with today, I can almost always say "been there, done that."

In the early 1990s – I was in my mid 20s and my life changed in two significant ways: I immigrated to Canada and I married my fiancé. Despite (and maybe because of) these life changing events, my dieting grew even more extreme. I weighed 110 pounds – too low for me, and felt drained by my obsession.

My doctor, concerned about my health, suggested that I enter an eating disorder program at Toronto General Hospital as an outpatient. I didn't particularly like being in the clinic – I wasn't "into" groups – but the hours I spent there did raise an interesting issue. Compared to the backgrounds of the other patients, most of who were victims of some form of abuse or other kind of trauma, mine appeared to be normal. "Why, then," I wondered, "Do I have this problem? What's my story?

To find it, I immersed myself in the subject reading dozens of books about eating disorders and personal growth. My goal was to find a pattern; every time I lost or gained weight, what were the surrounding incidents? Eventually, the answers starting coming to me; food, I began to understand, was not my problem.

As none of the dieticians nor doctors with whom I'd consulted seemed to realize, my dieting and eating patterns (and previously to some extent my tennis) were merely symptoms – they were my default coping mechanisms, ways to distract me from whatever real issues were bothering me. But more importantly they provided me with a sense of control in my life and an identity when clearly I did not feel that just being myself was enough. At least to me, it also seemed easier to manage than life.

Dieting alone wasn't an answer. But if I couldn't – or didn't diet, how was I going to control my weight? Identity issues once again unloosed me. If I was now no longer Lauren the tennis player *or* Lauren the dieter, *then* who was I?

The answers continued to evolve. One was to channel my love of sports and fitness into a more suitable career than the administrative work I did (unhappily) at the time. In 1997, I enrolled in a two-year program to earn my certification as a personal trainer. Ironically, I put on thirty pounds. Looking back, I understand my rationale: if I didn't succeed, I could always blame my weight, which, in terms of my ego, was far less threatening than admitting I wasn't a good trainer. Fortunately, clients continued to seek me out as a trainer, removing at least that insecurity.

Still, there *was* the weight. Like many dieters, I knew everything about nutrition – and nothing. To guide me through the thicket of true and false information, I enrolled in the Institute of Holistic Nutrition in Toronto. But the most important answers came as I continued my relentless self-scrutiny. From bitter experience, I now knew that all the fitness and nutritional principles in the world wouldn't help me if I didn't understand the forces that drove me to torment myself with food and dieting.

Putting together what I'd learned from these programs, my extensive ongoing research, as well as the hard, sometimes heartbreaking, lessons I'd learned from my own self-scrutiny, I finally realized that just being myself was enough. I did not have to be Lauren the tennis player or Lauren the dieter. I could just be myself, with my feelings, thoughts, ideas, values and morals.

This was the realization and self-acceptance that I had worked so hard to find and come to terms with and what ultimately changed my life forever. Finally I was comfortable and happy with whom I was and I did not need any external labels to define me. Then and only then was I equipped to develop principles that allowed me to sustain a healthy way of eating – and living –on which I still rely on today and which you will soon learn about.

As a result for most of the last ten years, I've maintained a healthy, lean weight (for me) of about 125 pounds. I don't go much below 125, nor do I swing above 130. Food and exercise no longer have the same power over my life that they once had. I've learned that living – staying fit and eating healthy – is always going to be somewhat of a struggle. There will always be struggles, challenges, growth and learning, and there is definitely no magic solution.

However, once you accept that idea, maintaining a healthy weight and even enjoying food, your life will be much less of a struggle. Even now, when I feel stress, I'm likely to fall back on my old patterns. Maybe I'll eat an extra chocolate bar, or, going to the other extreme, I'll cut calories or banish certain foods. But the difference is, now I understand why I am doing this and I don't indulge in these behaviours to the point of them being detrimental. My weight no longer fluctuates like the Dow Jones Index average. Instead I stay aware of what is happening in my life, how it is affecting me and then I deal with it, the best I can. It is that awareness, plus the habits I've taught myself and the knowledge about both mind and body I've acquired, that keeps destructive eating off my radar screen – at long last.

Beginning on page xxxii, you'll read ten basic principles of my program. Some of the principles are rather simple (and I give you easy ways to follow them): Watch your portions, balance your nutrients, and allow yourself treats. Principle 2, for example, suggests you keep a food journal. To this day I still walk around with my journal. If I'm going to a restaurant, I toss it in my purse. It's my compass. Will I ever give it up? Never! What's important to realize is that for anyone with a weight or food issue, diet is always going to require watching. It need not be an obsession, though; it can just be a factor in one's life, like diabetes, one that can be managed.

Further along, on page 60, I discuss barriers to eating successfully; these can be tricky. Consider triggers (which I define as particular moods or situations that lead us into emotional eating); twelve years ago, married but still trying to figure my way off of the dieting treadmill, I asked myself some difficult questions. One of those questions involved me identifying what my common triggers were at the time. It took me a while to figure this out, but eventually, with careful and honest reflection, I was able to identify many of my triggers, both past and present - they varied as much as my life did. For example, after being around certain people or situations I would almost always binge. I couldn't control whatever had upset me, but the eating was *my* problem. No one else was to blame. Once I took responsibility for my behaviour and developed a strategy to deal with it, these circumstances lost their power. I'd feel irritated afterwards, but I wouldn't binge. To insure that I wouldn't, I made certain that I did not have any tempting trigger foods waiting for me at home. More importantly, I learned to sit out the bad feelings. No amount of chocolate or cheesecake, I realized, was going to make those go away. Even anger no longer drove me back to my old patterns. I finally understood that other people's behaviours weren't always about me and I bounced back more quickly.

Sadly, in 2007 my husband and I parted after 13 years of marriage. By now I was definitely attuned to the knowledge and understanding that no amount of food would change how you feel and as a result I now went through a very different, yet similar experience. Fully aware of what I was doing, I decided that just this once in my life, I was consciously going to eat whatever I wanted, just because I wanted to. I knew I'd put on weight, and that I'd be unhappy about it but did it anyway. Sure enough, I gained about thirty pounds, and of course I wasn't totally happy about it. But, something had changed. Unlike in the past, I didn't beat myself up for the digression. The weight gain wasn't some sinister force that overwhelmed me; it was the consequence of a choice *I'd* made. I knew the origin of every pound I gained. I even kind of enjoyed the enterprise. At that point in my life, it was both what I wanted and needed to do. And yet, soon enough – and also by choice – I returned to my newly acquired, more satisfying way of eating and the weight disappeared.

So even today, knowing that a couple of pieces of chocolate wouldn't turn a bad day into a good one, I'll sometimes eat a couple anyway. Once in a while, I might even eat an entire bar. The difference is, I'm not expecting it to change my circumstances or how I feel and, I am completely aware of what I am doing; it's a very conscious choice, not an impulsive reaction. I will, however, most likely have a lighter dinner to make up for it but I definitely won't skip dinner and because I've followed the ten principles for healthy eating and living, and all the other advice laid out in this program, my body – and soul are better equipped to resist the onslaught.

I have one final piece of advice to impart before you start out on your journey. Throughout the book you'll notice quotes from famous thinkers (Nelson Mandela, Mahatma Gandhi, Eleanor Roosevelt) and some less famous ones (philosophers, authors, people I've encountered in everyday life). All of them speak to the topic of authenticity. If you want to eat like a whole person, you have to be a whole person. Now what does that mean? It doesn't mean you fly off to India or run an ultra- marathon or latch onto some extreme cause. It simply means you commit to finding and then being and accepting your authentic self. Let me dip back into my own story one last time.

Up until at least my late twenties, I did not live a completely authentic life. I studied for, and earned, my degree in elementary education because it was suitable and sensible, but I despised it. Today I teach fitness and nutrition; fields I chose because I love them and not because they were suitable or sensible or because I needed someone else's approval.

In 2001, my mother died after a long struggle with breast cancer. Her death had an enormous impact on me, one that I can only touch upon here. One small outcome, though, was that some years later (in 2008), I began volunteering for the Breast Cancer Foundation in my area. A few people close to me opposed my decision. They suggested I volunteer for an organization in which I was more likely to "meet someone nice" – in other words, a potential husband. They didn't understand that I wasn't volunteering because I had time on my hands, or because I wanted to meet people or because I had an agenda. My desire was only to contribute to a cause that had meaning for me. And in doing that, I was being authentic.

The false idols of weight and dieting will only keep you from being that person, and that's the real tragedy. In a way, the goal is circular. In order to eat well you need to live well, but in order to live well, you need to eat in a way that moves your life forward rather than holds you back.

We feed ourselves. It's one of the most basic and instinctive things we do. How we do it is connected to our behaviour, our health and our happiness. What does our well-being have to do with food; with exercise; with pH balance, metabolism, stress and all the other topics addressed in the following pages? The answer is "everything." In subsequent chapters, I tell you how these topics are all related. The underlying thesis is, of course (and you know this), is that fad diets don't work. What does work is a sane and healthy lifestyle. If you're ready, we can achieve it together.

INTRODUCTION

The last ten years have relieved me of the need to torture myself with food. I'm a comfortable size six and have the body of a person perhaps even ten years younger than I am. Better yet, I eat cheesecake (on occasion) – and enjoy it. So what's my secret? A few suggestions you've heard before – you probably know the basic rules of nutrition even if you don't follow them – and others that will allow you, in fact, to follow them.

Regardless of whether you have five pounds to lose or three hundred, whether you yo-yo, binge, graze, fast or starve, whether you are a couch potato or a competitive athlete (and I have all types among my clients); this book will give you not just everything you need to know about fitness and nutrition but the will to incorporate that knowledge into your life.

Diets don't work – they're seductive, they're fun – but let's face it, if they worked, a zillion dollar diet industry wouldn't be coaxing people to do ridiculous things of which no ethical doctor would approve. Changes in lifestyle, behaviour and attitude, however, do work. That's why this program – note I don't use the heinous word "diet" – is a way of life. It feeds you inside and out.

The heart and soul of this book are the 10 Change4Good Principles©. I developed them during the dozen years in which I've been a certified personal trainer and nutritionist as well as a lifestyle and wellness coach.

Before I explain them to you, I'd like to tell you about the many ways in which my approach differs from the many that take up squander space in magazines and air time on talk shows.

Unlike those diets, my program is not a trend, a fad, or the latest celebrity diet. You won't hear some movie star or celebrity boasting "I lost thirty pounds in thirty days!" and a year later see her thirty pounds heavier; having gained everything back. Instead, the ten principles reflect not only cutting edge science but the combined wisdom of my many years in the field as both a trainer and nutritionist and a (formerly) desperate and chronically unhappy dieter *(see My Story)*. Here is psychology, biology and a little bit of the salve that makes all systems go: *a little belief in yourself.*

Throughout my years of practice, I've trained a wide variety of clients, among them: Canada's world champion ballroom dancing team, nationally ranked swimmers and marathon runners. I've counselled entire hockey and soccer teams as well as age-ranked gymnasts.

In the civilian world, I treat doctors, lawyers and stockbrokers (talk about people under pressure), and brides (people under even *more* pressure); women who've just given birth, families and dozens of ordinary adults and teens.

In the corporate world, I've worked at AB Sciex, Ceridian, Bank of Montreal, Royal Bank of Canada, Mercedes-Benz, YMCA, the Running Room and Texas Instruments, to name just a few. My advice appears in print (magazines like More, iRun and Wedding Bells to name a few) and on both radio and television (I've been a featured speaker on both nationally and locally syndicated talk shows). Through all these experiences, the Change4Good program and ten principles evolved.

Crib Sheet: What Change4Good is and what it isn't:

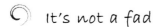 It's not a fad

It's based on principles that are meant to seep their way into your consciousness and change your ways of eating (and coping) for good. Unlike the chocolate or single-nutrient diet, the program is designed to sustain you over the long haul. Because its premise is based on long-standing principles of science and nutrition, it may evolve, but it won't disappear with tomorrow's headlines.

It's flexible

In my experience as a nutritionist, **rigid food plans don't work; flexible principles do.** Whether you're a Type A workaholic with no time to reduce a wad of kale into manageable portions or a stay-at-home type with too much time to stare into your soul (and the refrigerator); you can incorporate these principles. They're portable. They go with you on your honeymoon in Paris or your next business trip to Seoul. You won't need to abandon them simply because they don't mesh with your culture, background, weather or even your mood on any particular day. You maintain the ability to "season" them.

It's simple

No whacky ingredients, complicated rules or food shipments that can take a bigger chunk out of your budget than they take out of you. **Anyone, anywhere, can follow it.** But just because the program is simple, doesn't mean it's easy. When I first discovered you needed to drink one to two litres of water a day, I thought it was impossible. And for the first week or two, it was. Constantly, I was forgetting to drink my water ("Now where did I leave that water bottle?") Also, I was getting annoyed. I had to go to the bathroom constantly.

It wasn't until a few weeks into employing the principle that I realized I wasn't overeating as much as I had been during meals, I wasn't feeling as tired, and my skin was glowing. Suddenly, a simple habit that didn't seem so simple, after while became a much cherished part of my routine.

The beauty of the 10 Change4Good Principles© is that they work, if you work them. You see results. Now, while other people run around with their expensive and caloric frappe drinks, I have my low cost, no calorie water, which I carry in an earth-friendly way.

C) It's holistic

Old habits are hard to relinquish. You adopted them, at least initially, because they gave you pleasure. To replace them, even with those that you know will serve you better, requires both consistency and a kind of steely determination. That's why the program is holistic. **It takes into account the fact that change isn't just physical. It requires cooperation from the mind, the heart and the soul;** areas that too many trainers, dieticians, nutritionists and even doctors ignore.

Early in my practice, for example, I learned how ill-prepared people were to handle stress. They'd come in to see me Monday morning always with some excuse: "My mother was ill." "Relatives came to visit." "I was under terrible pressure at work." Well, problems, hardship, stress – they're facts of life. **If you decide to abandon your better habits every time a stressful situation emerges, you'll never get rid of your less helpful habits.** This is why I also include principles that focus on your entire well-being, not just those that can be weighed and measured. **Live well, eat well: the two go hand in hand.**

It trades perfectionism for consistency and moderation

The best way to achieve change is reasonably. Focus on small steps. Make one change that you know you can handle and the satisfaction you'll gain from employing it will spur you on to try another and another.

You'll be surprised how quickly small steps add up to large and meaningful change. And **don't expect yourself to be perfect.** *All or nothing attitudes with black and white thinking are lethal.* The ten principles coax you to be good, not perfect. They even build into them a little room for "cheating" (see Principle 8). Most importantly, **don't beat yourself if you fall short of your desired objective.** Instead, ask yourself: where did I mess up? Was there a reason? What can I do to improve? **Responsibility is different from guilt. Guilt isn't the way to succeed at healthy eating – at healthy anything.**

It's grounded in reality

The program keeps you accountable by giving you tools to measure and monitor your results. Are you in fact losing body fat rather than muscle; real inches and real pounds of body fat? Are you gaining muscle, both physical and mental? You don't want to get too attached to figures and numbers, but then you can't ignore them either. **Checking in with reality keeps you moving forward. It gives you cause to examine what is and isn't working and to take the actions you need to bring about the desired results.** Fantasy is fine but reality lasts.

It's cooperative

Unlike so many of the more bizarre plans out there, this one doesn't demand that you cut yourself off from your social circle. In fact, it works better if you involve your social circle in your program – *gently.* **Few people can achieve anything without support from the people around them.** Think of those in your life who will help you –

take long walks with you when you're stuck, urge you forward when you fall behind – *but choose wisely*. Even those we love sometimes have complicated reasons for not wanting us to succeed.

Since we tend to emulate the people around us, surround yourself with people whose qualities you admire. Share what you're doing with them. Ask for their support. And thank them by sharing what they've taught you with others whom you, too, can help. **Give love, get love: it's as true as any law of physics.**

And now, the principles – discussed at length in subsequent chapters, are listed below, accompanied by a few lines about each. Some are so simple you'll wince at how easy they seem; others may take a lifetime to perfect. Luckily, progress is apparent even from Day One. Remember, with principles instead of specific plans, you have the tools to change your life.

> *"Give a man a fish and you feed him for a day;*
> *teach a man to fish and you feed him for a lifetime."*
> ~Moshe ben-Maimon (Maimonides)

The Ten Essentials for Food, Fitness and the Good Life

1. **Cleanse your Mind;** Live Purposefully
2. **Set Goals;** Keep a Journal
3. **Identify Barriers;** Surmount Them
4. **Eat Well:** Lean Protein, Natural Carbohydrates and Healthy Fats at Each Meal
5. **Eat Often:** Four - Six Nutrient-Dense Meals/Snacks Each Day
6. **Read:** Those Tricky Food Labels
7. **Manage:** Food and Beverage Portions
8. **Practice:** Moderation; Follow the 90/10 Rule
9. **Drink:** One - Two Litres of Water Every Day
10. **Move:** Exercise at Least Thirty - Sixty Minutes Each Day

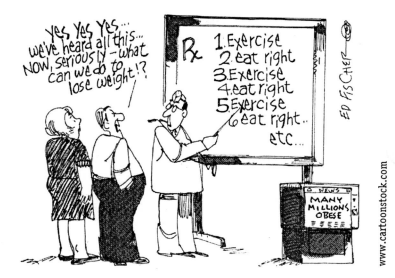

Principle 1 Cleanse your Mind; Live Purposefully

In a nutshell – be conscious. **The life you want will not happen by chance – you need to choose it** (to the extent that you can). You also need to be mindful. Pay attention to what you want and the strategies you are using to achieve it. Are they working? **In terms of food, be conscious of how much you are eating and why you are eating it.** You cannot be mindlessly eating while working, driving or watching a movie. During workouts, be conscious of every muscle you use and why. If you know that contracting your glutes will give you a firmer butt, you'll do it with conviction instead of acting as if it were drudgery. Chapter ONE shows you how to implement this principle in other areas of your life.

Principle 2 Set Goals: *Keep a Journal*

Unless you set goals, you aren't likely to achieve them. Chapter TWO helps with the hard part, figuring out exactly what goals you want to set. In terms of food and exercise, writing a journal helps. Who wants to keep a journal especially when they're veering off track? Not you. Do it anyway. Keeping a record of what you eat, how you feel and how much you're exercising is one of the factors that correlate most strongly with success of the outcome. It tethers you to reality so that when an emotional situation comes up, you don't have to panic and regress. **You have a plan – in writing. Use it. Remember, failing to plan is planning to fail.**

Principle 3 Identify Barriers; Surmount Them

Ups and downs – they're true of life; not just of your weight. **The more skilled we become at dealing with the tough stuff, including the tough stuff of our own making, the better we will be able to stay on track.** Chapter THREE (and others) will help you to identify barriers and give you tools with which to manage. **The goal is for you to manage these obstacles – not let them manage you.**

Principle 4 Eat Well: Lean Protein, Natural Carbohydrates and Healthy Fats at Each Meal

It's so logical but so hard for some of us. Start with breakfast. Does it have all three of those elements? A carb-laden muffin may be easier but it won't stay with you for more than an hour after you eat it, and it won't look as good inside your clothes.

Combine lean protein, natural carbohydrates and healthy fats in the right proportion, as Chapter FOUR advises, and all sorts of lovely things will happen. Among them: you'll slow digestion, which will keep your blood glucose level stable, release less insulin and cause less fat to be stored. **Your moods and energy won't ricochet**, which, whether you realize it or not, they do following coffee and a muffin.

Principle 5 Eat Often: Four - Six Nutrient-Dense Meals/Snacks Each Day

Begin within an hour or two of waking. Keep meals and snacks approximately three hours apart throughout the rest of the day. Have your last meal or snack at least two hours before bedtime. Eating regularly will keep your body healthy and you functioning optimally. Finally, don't eat an hour before and after exercise - this will help maximize fat burning both during and after your workout.

As for quality, healthy food is more user-friendly. Junk food stimulates your appetite for (guess what) more junk food. Junk food, as Chapter FOUR will explore, gives you calories but not the nutrition you need. It's like putting pop in the gas tank of your car. The tank may be full, but the car will never move. And if you need any more information to convince you: your skin, your hair, your teeth – all of you – will be getting the essential nutrients they need to function optimally, when you eat healthy.

Principle 6 Read: Those Tricky Food Labels

People put so much effort into researching television screens, cell phones and cars before they buy them, but when it comes to their bodies, of which each person only has one, some people hardly pay attention. On the other hand, manufacturers don't make it easy for people to know, since packages that scream "healthy," or "low-fat" may not be telling the whole story. **Learning to read food labels – and see beyond the hype – is critical to your ability to shop intelligently.** You don't have to stand in the supermarket aisle as if it were a museum. Learning a few basic rules laid out in Chapter SIX will help you navigate your way through all the hieroglyphics and guide you to the good stuff wherever you are.

Principle 7 Manage: Food and Beverage Portions

A client eats a bowl of popcorn every night. What a shock for her to discover that she was actually eating not one or two but three serving sizes as listed on the package. It didn't stop her from eating popcorn as her late night snack, but now that she saw how much she was consuming, she began to eat less.

Certainly it's no longer breaking news that portion sizes and even utensils have mutated during the last decade. **Supersizing has distorted our perception of what a regular serving of food should be with the result that most people are consuming more calories than they can burn off even if they are active.** The trick is learning to eat until you're somewhat satisfied – but not full to the point of discomfort. "Ah, if only I could do that," you're telling yourself. Don't worry – listening to your body is so difficult that it's not merely a skill; it's an art. Chapter SEVEN will help you acquire it.

Principle 8 Practice: Moderation; Follow the 90/10 Rule

This maxim applies to how you approach and follow this program as well. In other words, I'm going to order you to occasionally eat a donut (or whatever your treat-of-choice may be). Ninety percent of the time you will follow the 10 Change4Good Principles© and ten percent of the time you allow yourself leeway – both in terms of your nutritional intake and your exercise regimen. Ten percent however doesn't mean twenty. Don't think: "I want another donut." Think: "Look, I'm thin and fit and healthy AND I can have **one** donut." There will be more on how to apply this principle (the most popular one in the program) in Chapter EIGHT.

Principle 9 Drink: One - Two Litres of Water Every Day

Bodies are bones and flesh but mostly, they're plain old H_2O – approximately sixty percent. Not surprisingly, water regulates all of our functions. It affects weight, regularity, bloating and energy. **Start your day with a glass of warm water and lemon.** The warm water stimulates your colon; while the lemon does lovely things for your liver (see Chapter NINE). The shocking fact is a large percentage of people walk around partially dehydrated. If you're thirsty, that's a sign that you already are dehydrated.

Principle 10 Move: Exercise at Least Thirty - Sixty Minutes Each Day

Diet alone doesn't work (see My Story). **You need exercise as well. Physical activity burns calories, increases metabolic rate and energy, and relieves stress,** all illustrated in Chapter TEN. And those hours do not have to be unpleasant. Dance your heart out. Run or power walk with a friend. Find those activities that you like so well that you'll want to do them. Keep in mind the difference between an active lifestyle and exercising. You want both.

An active lifestyle means taking the stairs instead of the elevator, parking your car at the furthest entrance from the mall, getting off the subway one stop sooner than you have to, walking the golf course instead of taking the golf cart – that sort of thing.

Exercise is structured – you have a program, a plan of progression, you participate at a higher intensity level but you also have fun. A close friend began working out at the gym a few months after her father died. It reduced her jeans size but more important, it helped her get through that difficult transition. Another trained and entered fitness competitions to overcome depression. Exercise is an elixir – use it. **Aim for a minimum of five hours per week.**

To live and breathe these principles so that they become instinctual, download multiple copies of them at www.change4good.ca. Plaster copies everywhere: in your car, office, desk and refrigerator. Heed them – and soon enough they'll be a part of who you are.

Final send-off tips:

1. **Don't get overwhelmed.** There's a lot of information in the remaining chapters. You might want to read a chapter a week, or a chapter a month. Move at your own pace.

2. **There is no correct order in which to implement the principles or even read the chapters.** I've written them in an order that makes sense to me. Read Chapter TEN first if metabolism and fitness are what excites you. Or Chapter THREE, if you want to figure out the obstacles before you encounter them. Just keep in mind that to achieve the best outcome, ultimately, you'll have to embrace all the ten principles.

3. **Each chapter contains Change4Good Action Steps, Tools and a "Remember This" tip.** Action steps help you use the principles; the tools help you complete the action steps. The "Remember This" tip at the end of each chapter is not a nag, just a friendly reminder to keep you on track all day, through good moments and bad.   Look for the following icons which will indicate:

 Action Steps   **Tools** – all tools can be downloaded at **www.change4good.ca**

 "Remember This"

So remember, don't just read this book. Live it.

"Be the change you want to see in the world."
~Mahatma Gandhi

CHANGE4GOOD

The Ten Essentials for Food, Fitness and the Good Life

Change Your Mind

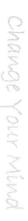

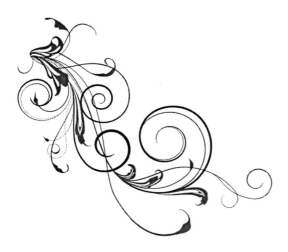

MIND YOUR BODY

This chapter is about the nutrients you give your soul.

Principle **1** Cleanse your Mind; *Live Purposefully*

Change begins in the mind, the heart and the soul, mysterious quarters that clients and even some practitioners tend to ignore. In those areas reside the potential for change. Chapter ONE gives you the nudge you need to live not like you're waiting for your life to happen but as if it were – and is – happening. Dress rehearsal over. Curtains up. Live now.

> **"Change your thoughts and you change your world."**
> ~Norman Vincent Peale, Minister and Author of,
> "The Power of Positive Thinking."

Welcome to the start of eating – and living – sanely. This chapter is about what needs to happen to your insides in order for your outsides to change for the better. Mostly, we'll center on your thoughts. **It's a frightening concept but you actually do have the power to achieve a good deal of what you want -- if you are willing to relinquish old beliefs that no longer serve you.** After years of studying how people change – and experiencing extraordinary change in my own life as well – I've noted the emergence of certain key agents of change.

 Be Crystal Clear About What You Want

Visualize it. See it. Focus on it in your mind.

For example: One summer I trained with an Olympic Gold Medalist athlete. One routine required me to jump hurdles. They weren't very high hurdles but they *were* hurdles. No matter what I did, I couldn't clear all the bars. On the night before one of our practice sessions, I lay in bed, envisioning myself clearing hurdle after hurdle. How glorious it felt. The next day, astonishing both the trainer and myself, I cleared every one. "Wow," he said, "yesterday you could hardly clear one and today, you're clearing all of them."

How did this happen? Although there are numerous theories as to the exact mechanism that causes visualization to work, a common explanation is that during visualization you physiologically create neural patterns in your brain as if you had physically performed an action and in so doing you train your mind to teach your muscles what to do. Virtually all studies provide sufficient reliable evidence that there is not only improved motor performance and therefore improved athletic performance but also greater mental toughness and confidence.

Visualization can also help you psychologically in the same way rehearsing does: it helps you manage the emotional stress that otherwise might "manage" you.

Take a situation involving food. Envision yourself at a high-powered business conference. *My, those breakfast pastries look tempting – just the thing to soothe my anxiety.* But if you rehearse reaching for the fruit basket, you might actually reach for it instead.

Visualization also works in more complicated situations.

After my mother died, I didn't see how I would get through her funeral. I'm the kind of person who cries even when saying goodbye to a friend. As the day approached, I pictured over and over again how it would unfold. The day unfolded as I had visualized it, this was no surprise as funerals were all conducted in the same way in Cape Town. What was astounding was that my emotions, under the circumstances, were remarkably controlled. It was as if I had been through this a hundred times before. My pain wasn't that raw. And in retrospect, I *had* been through it a hundred times before – in my head. I understood then how visualization can affect our response.

Our subconscious works in images. For this reason, I often recommend **Vision Boards** to clients. Even if you aren't especially visual, give it a shot. Take a poster board and fill it with pictures that accurately depict something that you want and that generates strong positive emotions in you (the front door of the lovely brownstone you'd like to buy; a gorgeous runner jogging over rough terrain). Place the mural where you'll see it every day.

A friend of mine pasted a picture of the Mini Cooper she longed for but couldn't afford, on a vision board in her bedroom. She even pasted a picture of her face on the windshield. After gazing at it long enough and taking action by making some changes in her lifestyle, she saved enough money to buy one. She actually achieved her desired end. If you're still skeptical, think of visualization as a prolonged (and less expensive) form of hypnosis.

 ## Want it, and Want it Badly

Sure some of you, anyway, may want to run the elite Boston Marathon – see yourself in a runner's magazine, shimmering medals dangling from your heaving chest. But do you want it badly enough to wake up two hours earlier, six days a week, to train? Probably not, which is why thousands rather than millions of people actually run the Boston Marathon.

If you don't want to achieve an outcome badly enough to endure the pain and effort required, it's better to know that up front. Otherwise, you'll waste precious energy pursuing what you don't really want that badly.

A good test is to ask yourself, "What do I need to do to achieve this goal?" "Am I willing to do this?" If the answer is yes, you're ready to start. If the answer is no, find a goal that motivates you so strongly that you *are* willing to do what it takes to achieve it.

 ## Uncover What Holds You Back

Sometimes you aren't willing to do what it takes to achieve a particular goal because of fear: you aren't convinced that you'll really be able to achieve it. Examine that fear. Is it reality?

Recently I saw a client who was convinced she couldn't stick to her personal Change4Good food plan we'd worked out. When I asked her why, she explained that her job had changed; she was travelling more and under too much pressure to think about what she ate. I doubted that this was the reason.

Working the tools of the program, I showed her how she could – easily – overcome what she thought were insurmountable obstacles – the lack of time, the constant eating out, the pressure – and eat in a way that would actually increase her ability to perform. If you take the time to break it down and work it out, usually there is a solution. Chapter THREE talks in greater detail about obstacles and how to overcome them.

 Match Your Actions with Your Goals

I worked with a runner who said she wanted to lose twenty pounds. "But I'm addicted to sugar; I love ketchup, and I won't give up aspartame." I was tempted to say, "Okay – see you later." After all, I'm not a miracle-worker. Instead, I coaxed her to re-frame the situation. "Can you give up aspartame, for example, just for one day?" I asked. You'd be surprised how quickly one day turns into five which turns into a whole year and suddenly, you're living aspartame-free.

Another client also wanted to lose twenty to thirty pounds. (Doesn't everyone?) Unfortunately, she and her friends liked to hang out and smoke marijuana, which of course gave them the munchies. "Do you want to lose the twenty pounds badly enough to give up smoking pot?" I asked, because only she could answer that question.

This is what psychology calls living intentionally. Are your actions consistent with your goals? *If you want to go anywhere, make sure your mind and your feet are in agreement.*

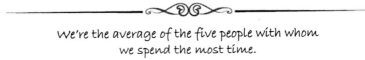 *Pay Attention to Peer Influence*

Research conducted by the late Jim Rohn, the legendary motivational speaker (his students included, among others, Jack Canfield of the "Chicken Soup®" series fame); suggests that, "We're the average of the five people with whom we spend the most time."[1] Do you complain a lot? Chances are your friends and loved ones complain a lot as well. Does food seem to be the center of all your activities? Chances are your friends punctuate every occasion with a meal.

The implications are obvious: if you want to feel better, hang around with people whose outlook is more constructive; if you want to lose weight, find a friend whose idea of a good time is a movie or, heaven forbid, a hike. **Surround yourself with people who exemplify the changes you want to see in yourself.**

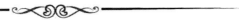

We're the average of the five people with whom we spend the most time.

To check yourself, Rohn suggests you ask yourself certain fundamental questions:

- *"Who am I around?"*
- *"What are they doing to me?"*
- *"What have they got me reading?"*
- *"What have they got me saying?"*
- *"Where do they have me going?"*
- *"What do they have me thinking?"*
- *"And most important, what do they have me becoming?"*
- *Then ask yourself the big question: "Is that okay?"*

"Your life does not get better by chance, it gets better by change."[2]

For ten years, I was friends with a woman who constantly complained about two topics: her weight and her boyfriend. I saw how drained I was after talking with her for even half an hour. You want to be a good friend, but allowing someone to perpetuate their anxiety by replaying it constantly doesn't help either of you.

Even the most resolved individual often yields in the face of peer pressure and influence. In Chapter SEVEN, we're going to discuss portion control in detail. But **looking at how and with whom you eat is almost more important than knowing how much to eat.**

Brian Wansink, an author and director of the Food and Brand Lab at Cornell University, has spent well over a decade studying what influences why we eat, how much we eat and how frequently we eat. He finds that when it comes to food, our mind is out-manoeuvred by external stimuli. We may know intellectually about portion control, for example, and still act in ways that utterly contradict that information.

Obviously, other factors are at work. Among them, Wansink's work suggests, are what the people around us eat and the amount and speed with which they eat it.[3] Hence, more justification for scrutinizing your peers, as discussed in Chapter THREE, when you're trying to adopt a healthier lifestyle.

I'm as good as any illustration of Wansink's research. Even with all I know about nutrition, I tend to make poorer choices when I eat out with friends who aren't as health conscious as I am.

"It is easier to change your environment than to try to outsmart your brain when it comes to situations around food."[4]

Change4Good Attitude GPS©

The following exercise, using the Change4Good Attitude GPS© (stands for Global Positioning System or, for our purposes, **Guide to Personal Success**), is a great tool to help you navigate your wisest course. (You'll see this exercise repeated in the book using a Behaviour, Nutrition and Fitness GPS.)

I've listed key aspects related to attitude that may need adjusting– but feel free to improvise and add your own:

◯ Realistic

> Do you see things the way they really are or do you tend to either see things the way you want them to be or the way you fear they could be?

◯ Optimistic

> Are you generally positive about life or even what you can salvage from a bad situation or do you tend to see the worst no matter how bad or good the situation?

◯ Self-Aware

> Do you understand, to some extent, your feelings? Why you have them and how they affect your life and the lives of those around you? Do you know your strengths and weaknesses and how to use them to your best advantage? Example: You have excellent time management skills, which ensure that you generally complete all your plans.

Constructive Dialogue with Self or Others

What is the little voice in your head saying most of the time? Is it positive and encouraging or negative and berating? Using realistic positive affirmations is a great way to change self-talk and your actions as well. For example, has saying "I'm so fat" all the time helped you stop overeating? I didn't think so.

But if you replace it, for example, with "I am getting healthier with every nutritious meal I have" then almost (but not quite) magically, you'll actually do what it takes to become that healthier being.

Flexible

Are you able to adjust how you think, act and feel when circumstances dictate or are you rigid even to your own detriment?

Solution Rather than Problem Oriented

Are you able to solve problems in a creative and positive way or do you get stuck or see the problem as unsolvable?

Assertive (but nicely)

Are you able to express and defend your opinions with grace; without being confrontational?

⟲ *Able to Manage Stress*

Can you pause, get a grip and reflect under pressure or do you react impulsively?

⟲ *Empathetic*

Are you able to put yourself in someone else's shoes? Do you place sufficient value on helping and serving others? In conflict situations, can you conceive of win/win solutions rather than ones that are win/lose?

All these qualities will affect how well you implement the other nine Change4Good Principles©. Therefore, take some time to carefully examine your attitude and identify what aspects of your way of thinking most needs to be changed. Obviously, you can't "cleanse" your toxic attitudes over night, but the longest journey, as you surely know, begins with a single step. The following exercise will help you take the journey.

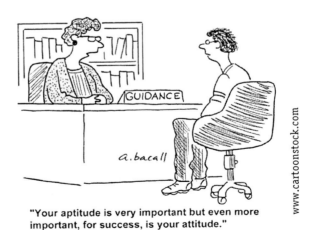

GUIDANCE

a.bacall

www.cartoonstock.com

"Your aptitude is very important but even more important, for success, is your attitude."

Change4Good Attitude GPS©

What to do:

1. Using the Change4Good Attitude GPS© rate your level of satisfaction for each separate area between zero and ten (ten being complete satisfaction; zero being none).

2. Place one dot (per segment) opposite the number that best represents your level of satisfaction.

3. Connect the dots to create a "circle" within the circle. **Unless you're consistently happy or miserable in every area of your life, the circle-within-the-circle is bound to be asymmetrical.**

Below is an example of a completed Change4Good Attitude GPS©

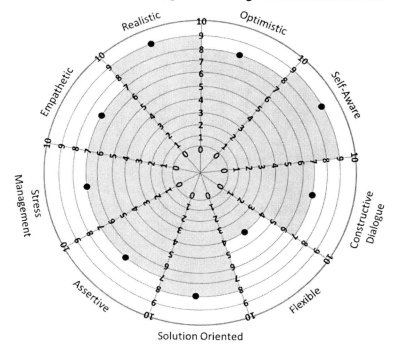

Your Change4Good Attitude GPS©

Now use the blank Change4Good Attitude GPS© below to
complete yours. You can also download it at
www.change4good.ca.

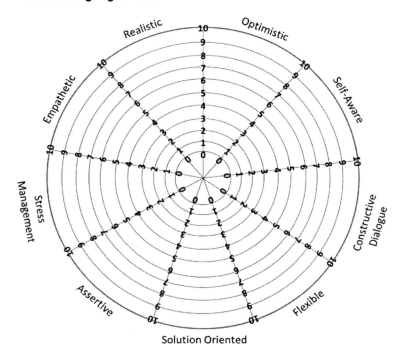

Solution Oriented

Now consider the following:

1. **How large is your circle?** Bigger is better.
2. **How symmetrical is it?** Your goal is to push everything to
   the outer rim, to have the largest, roundest circle.
3. **Where does your circle dip toward the center? The dips
   indicate the areas you most need to address?** These areas
   will form the basis of your "goals" in Chapter TWO. In the
   meantime, let's examine in more detail ways in which you
   can push each mini-arc outward.

Focus On the Solution

It is common wisdom that if you focus on the problem, the problem grows. If you focus on the solution, the solution grows. The logic of this maxim is apparent. If you continually complain about being fat, you'll feel unhappy. Unhappiness creates stress. Stress creates the need to escape. M&Ms are an escape.

Complain about your situation enough and you'll find yourself eating foods for the wrong reasons. If, however, you focus on a solution, on wanting to become more fit, and on the way to achieve it (four to six nutritious meals/snacks a day, thirty to sixty minutes exercise a day etc.); you might find yourself browsing through running magazines. Maybe you'll jog home from work. Endorphins will kick in (see Chapter TEN). You'll feel inspired. M&Ms? They most likely won't even enter your mind.

Focus on the problem, the problem grows.
Focus on the solution, the solution grows.

One example from my life where focussing on the solution worked really well for me was when I wanted to buy a condominium. I loved the condominium I was renting; only financially, I knew it wasn't a wise long-term proposition. I fussed a bit, but then I acted. I carefully analyzed the situation, coming up with the three criteria that mattered most to me (size, style and location).

I then conveyed that information to my realtor. Eventually, the perfect condominium appeared. Ready and armed, I acted and it's now my lovely home. Whether it appeared because I had done my homework and was ready, well, who knows? But it's amazing how the right solutions come when we're ready for them (meaning we've put in the work).

Conversely, one area of my Attitude GPS that tends to dip to the center is flexibility. I think back to how many times I turned down invitations to go out with friends, go on weekend getaways with my ex-husband because I was on a diet and would only eat food that I had prepared and bought or because the trip would disrupt my workout routine. What a loss on my part. If only I had known then about the 10 Change4Good Principles©; part of whose beauty is that they're flexible.

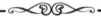

*No plan you do should require you to be so
rigid that you're missing out on life.*

Avoid Blame

How nice to blame our spouse, our parents, our boss, our metabolism, our "ex" – the world – for everything wrong in our lives. It requires no effort and fills us with a feeling of, well, delicious outrage. I'm sorry to tell you but blame isn't constructive. It makes you feel like a victim and who wants to be that? **Better to correct a situation where you can and accept those situations that you cannot change.** But no matter what you do, avoid the inertia that is the progeny of blame.

For many years, I had a friend who made me ⌐
unimportant. If, hypothetically we were stand.
the rain and I said it was raining, she'd disagre〈
with me. If anyone else said it was raining well
then, it was raining. She was important to me foı
other reasons, which is why I maintained the
friendship.

Still, I often reacted to the feelings of worthlessness
I experienced when I was with her by overeating.
Eventually, I saw my error. She wasn't going to
change but that didn't mean I couldn't. I made a
careful pact with myself not to wither at her lack of
regard for me. Rather than get angry or worse –
internalize her opinion of me – I simply reminded
myself, "That's her problem, not mine." Now I say
what I think and detach myself from her reaction.
Easy? No. Effective? Absolutely!

Get Honest, Be Honest, Stay Honest

Sometimes, we actually prefer the problem we know to
one we fear. An example: a former co-worker of mine,
who was obese, complained bitterly about her sleep
apnea. It's a known fact that sleep apnea is connected to
being overweight. The fact that she chose not to work on
her weight problem, instead suggests that she feared
giving up the comfort of her food more than she did the
sleep apnea. If she could acknowledge that problem, she
might rouse the strength within herself to tackle her
problem.

**When we're stuck, like my former co-worker was, it's
usually because there's a payoff in being stuck.** We may
not know what the payoff is, but it's there.

For this reason, **it's really important to spend the time to know yourself. And to do this, you must be honest.** Ask yourself: what's the payoff in holding on to this problem? And more importantly, what's the fear I have in letting it go?

As in the previous example, the answers are usually obvious; it's just that we aren't willing to see them.

- Be open to advice.
- Listen to trusted friends.
- Pay attention to your fears – they usually explain the source of your resistance.

Trust Your Inner Voice

Use your intuition (fancy way of saying live authentically). Granted, intuition is a tricky concept. It isn't quite the same as desire or want. You want a frosty milkshake. Your intuition says it might not be such a good idea. Desire is exciting. Intuition is more serene. Desire shouts. Intuition whispers. Desire often overrides fear, but fear often stands in the way of intuition.

I was afraid and of course sad to end my marriage – at the time, family and many friends opposed it – but I did it anyway. I listened to my intuition and made what for me was although the hard choice, the right choice. Fear and pressure often block us from hearing our intuition.

Two years ago, I received an invitation to celebrate the Bat Mitzvah of a friend's son at a sit-down luncheon. Instinctively, I knew I didn't want to go alone and didn't have anyone appropriate to take. My friend, I knew, didn't have friends who weren't part of a couple. "But I'll put you with great people," she coaxed. It would've been easier to say 'yes' and please my friend, but intuition – or past experience – told me I shouldn't. When I had been in similar situations in the past, I paid the price, often by overeating. This time, I attended the religious service and sent a gift, but didn't attend the luncheon. Instead, I spent a perfectly delightful afternoon elsewhere. **It's a powerful feeling to allow yourself to be authentic.**

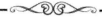

Desire is exciting – intuition is more serene.
Desire shouts – intuition whispers.
Desire often overrides fear,
But fear often stands in the way of intuition.

Accentuate the Positive

Earlier in the chapter we quoted Norman Vincent Peale, on the benefits of positive thinking. The field of Neuro-Linguistic Programming suggests a scientific underpinning for Peale's thesis.

What you say (even to yourself), it turns out, isn't always what your brain hears. For example, if you say to yourself, "I won't overeat," the brain hears "overeat, I won't." That's because the brain hears positive words first. Tell your child "don't spill the milk," and his brain will hear "spill the milk, don't." Better to say "hold your glass carefully" or even "keep your glass of milk steady." As a society, we tend to speak in negative terms. Don't you?

Look for Lessons

Whether you believe that everything in life happens for a reason or not, believing it does, helps. When events don't turn out the way we want them to, we naturally despair. Some of us even wallow in the misery that has befallen us. And some misery really is miserable. At least regarding the everyday traumas of living, it's often good to retain humility.

Ask yourself, "How do I know that what is happening to me is necessarily so negative. Maybe I wasn't meant to get that apartment (guy, dress or promotion) because a better one awaits me." Regarding relationships, especially, I know sometimes they don't work out because we still have some lessons to learn, either about ourselves or relationships in general. **Learn from your situation. It may serve you in the future in ways you can't even begin to realize now.**

Learn From Your Gaffes

Easier said than done, I know. But learning from life's lessons is inevitable, if you practice Principle 1; which is another way of telling you to remain teachable. Pay attention to your life. See what it has to teach you. Even when you don't understand why an event is happening, trust that you will in the future if you remain aware. And how do you remain aware? Let's recap:

- Be honest; examine a painful or positive event in retrospect and see what lesson you can draw from it.
- When a similar situation appears, notice how much easier it will be for you to handle. Notice how much less of a storm it unleashes inside you.

- Finally, as past experience crystallizes inside you, you'll develop intuition; you'll learn to listen to that small voice inside you even before a situation fully develops.

Pay attention to your life—
See what it has to teach you.

Fortunately, life gives us plenty of opportunities to learn tough lessons. In fact, until you learn the lessons you are meant to learn, it will seem as if similar situations keep presenting themselves. And once you're able to learn from those situations, the universe will stop sending them to you. **You'll become a trained athlete at handling emotional stress.**

And learn we do. Two years ago, I was worried about my finances. An acquaintance told me about a business scheme in which I could make more money in a week than I made in a month. Everything in my being (the little voice in my head) told me not to invest in the scheme. Still, I didn't listen. Naturally, I lost most of the money. I paid a high price for not listening but at least I learned from my past mistake.

Eventually, when confronted with a similar offer, I easily refused. If you find yourself making the same errors repeatedly, then go back to the subheading in this chapter entitled "Get Honest, Be Honest, Stay Honest." Obviously you're getting something from the action that's serving a purpose, however high the price.

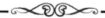 *Monitor Your Thoughts and Actions*

They actually affect your health. Consider what happens when you have a stressful thought. You feel a pounding in your chest – inside, your heart is beating more rapidly. But stress causes other changes inside you. Every thought or feeling you have corresponds to a chemical or physical change. Let's say you feel your heart pounding because of stress. Stress causes other chemical reactions as well. It causes a release of cortisol (or hydrocortisone), a steroid hormone produced by the adrenal gland. Cortisol causes an increase in your appetite; it also causes your body to store fat. **Regardless of whether the stress is perceived or real, whether your body or your mind experience stress, stress produces the same physiological effect.**

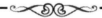

Toxic thoughts affect more than our behaviour. They actually affect our health. Every thought or feeling we have corresponds to a chemical or physical change.

"Happiness is when what you think, what you say, and what you do are in harmony."
~Mahatma Gandhi

So far, my approach has been: **change your thoughts and you'll change your actions as well.** But changing your actions (and environment) sometimes has an equally healthful effect on your mind. This is good news because some people find it easier to change their actions than to change their minds. We absolutely do have the ability to change our brain by changing our behaviour. So many sources have shown that the structure of our brain actually changes based on how be behave day to day.

This means that we can undo old patterns and develop new and more constructive ones. In terms of habits, I have found with my clients that it takes *at least* three to four weeks for changes to occur; so be patient and realize some habits are harder to unlearn and will take longer to become a part of your unconscious.

Let's say, just because I tell you to do it, you make your kitchen nutrition-friendly (you'll see how in Chapter SIX). You'll get rid of the processed food and stock up on whole grains and healthy beverages and snacks. Your attitude hasn't changed – you still would rather eat a packet of gummies than an orange – but your surroundings have.

Now, let's say it's ten o'clock at night and you have a yen for the gummies. The only way you can get them is to put on your parka and drive (in the cold) to the nearest convenience store; where who knows if they will even have them. *Suddenly, the oranges in the bowl on the counter start to look more appealing.* You try one, and because part of the Change4Good program involves buying the loveliest whole foods you can, you discover that in fact, the orange is remarkably sweet and juicy. You get into eating oranges. Maybe you try other healthy foods. Maybe your weight goes down. Maybe your friends start to notice – and tell you – how good you look.

Suddenly you feel empowered to make other changes that you longed to make; changes that have nothing to do with food, like upgrading your skills or finding a better job or mate or group of girlfriends. **Losing unnecessary weight is not just about a number on the scale, it's also about how it makes you feel about yourself.** And feeling confident and bold and successful is critical.

Just the other day, I spoke to a client who said that she wanted to try the Change4Good program, but was apprehensive. "I know if I don't eat sugar, I'll be hungry for it." In fact, the opposite is true. When you reduce your intake of simple sugars, your craving for them decreases. A perfect example of how **changing the way you act changes what goes on in your mind and body.**

Un-Multi Task

Be completely present and focussed in whatever you do. To accomplish this, reduce as much as possible and when appropriate, the amount of stimuli (TV, music, noise) you are exposed to. This will improve productivity and will also ensure you truly experience every part of your life without taking anything for granted.

Annually I go back to South Africa, where I grew up, to visit my family. We all long to spend time together, as it only happens once a year. I especially cherish the time with my young nephew and nieces. The reason I have the most incredible memories of these visits that will remain with me forever, is because when I am with my family, I am truly present in the moment and giving them 100% of my attention. This was not always the case. I used to be a multi-tasker, playing with them, checking emails on my BlackBerry® and who knows what else, all at the same time. Until I realized how I was cheating everyone by not being present and focused. This is true of life as well; when you do a million things at once, barely any stay with you.

Finally, in conclusion, here are some additional key factors for personal well-being:

Be Authentic

Live honestly by being true to yourself. See things the way they really are and always maintain a positive attitude.

Take Action

Know what you want to do and don't be afraid to pursue it. Remember that when you step out of your comfort zone is when you grow and reap the greatest rewards. Know the legacy you wish to leave behind and create it.

> "We gain strength, and courage, and confidence by each experience in which we really stop to look fear in the face... we must do that which we think we cannot."
> ~Eleanor Roosevelt

Be Grateful

The patriarchs of almost every religion espouse this attitude and you can understand why. By the time you finish listing all that you are grateful for in your life, *you will feel grateful*. **Gratitude leads to humility and acceptance; two ingredients for a happy life.**

Be Kind

It is so easy to pay someone a compliment, let someone into your lane of traffic. You will make someone else feel good, including yourself.

Finally, Have Fun

Life is too short not to take time to enjoy the company of good friends, be in nature or undertake whatever rejuvenates and relaxes you. Make this a regular priority in your life.

CHANGE4GOOD – ACTION STEPS

- Start implementing Principle 1 - Cleanse your Mind; Live Purposefully.

- Create your Vision Board.

- Complete your Change4Good Attitude GPS©.

- Develop a positive affirmation for yourself. For example: "I am getting healthier with every meal I have, I feel more energetic every day, I love drinking water." Change it as frequently as you need to, but always have one.

 ## TOOLS

- Change4Good Attitude GPS©

REMEMBER THIS

- How you think affects how you act; ask yourself, are my thoughts and behaviours constructive?

Change Your Behaviours

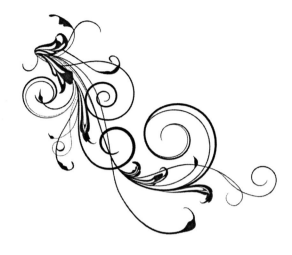

Chapter **TWO**

Change Your Behaviours

ON YOU MARK, GET SET, GOAL

Goals give you a place to go; strategies give you a way to get there. In this chapter, you get down to basics. Name your goals. Write them in your journal. I'll help you figure out a way to achieve them.

Principle **2** Set Goals; Keep a Journal

A small effort that pays off big-time is setting goals, writing them down and then monitoring your progress at pursuing them. Knowing where you want to end up and writing it all down keeps you aware and focused. And watch: soon your goals will be a reality and your journal will become your best friend. You'll be lost without it.

> "We are what we repeatedly do.
> Excellence then, is not an act, but a habit."
> ~Aristotle, Greek Philosopher

Having completed your Change4Good Attitude GPS© in the previous chapter, you're aware of ways of thinking that you want to improve. Let's translate the resultant goals – to think more constructively, for example – as well as other desires you may harbour into specific goals.

- Some of those goals will be large (improving your relationship with your sister).
- Some will be abstract (feeling better about yourself in general).
- Some will be very specific and measurable, involving the size of your hips and waist or the amount of exercise you do every week.

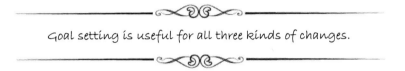

Goal setting is useful for all three kinds of changes.

GOAL SETTING

- Take time to really think about what you (not what your friends, relatives or parents) want to achieve, and why.

- Crystallize those desires into concrete goals (I want to feel good about myself; I want to have more stamina, I want to get along with my sister).

- Set a long term goal (what you'd ultimately like to achieve) as well as short term or weekly goals (your means of getting there).

- Pair each goal with a strategy for achieving it.

Let's talk about goals for a moment. There are two varieties: **behaviour-based** and **outcome-based.**

Behaviour Goals: These are actions you can directly control, such as eating 4-6 small meals per day. The 10 Principles, by the way, are all behaviour-based; they're all within your control. Some, such as drinking water more frequently, are easier to control than others (empathize, even when dealing with an annoying relative).

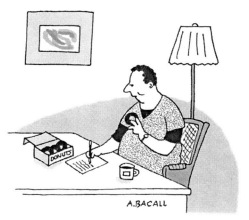

I resolve to drive past a gym at least twice a week."

A.BACALL

www.cartoonstock.com

Outcome Goals: These are the results of behaviour goals but not as directly within your control. You can eat 4-6 small meals a day during a particular week; you can't say with as much certainty how much weight that behaviour will cause you to lose. A mix of factors determines the outcome. Odds are, however, if you stick to your strategy, you'll get to your goal. It's just not always possible to predict when. Therefore, it is best to concentrate on behaviour goals rather than outcome goals. Ask yourself: am I eating 4-6 small but healthy meals each day? Not, "Am I losing weight this minute, hour or day?" Rest assured: as long as you follow the 10 Change4Good Principles© consistently, you'll eventually achieve the goal.

The short term behaviour goals you set need to be maintained for the long term in order to reach your ultimate outcome goal. Each week (or as you feel comfortable) you will add new short term goals to your lifestyle. As you maintain these new behaviours you will be developing a new lifestyle for yourself; one that will undoubtedly translate into achieving your long term outcome goal.

For example: This week, I want to eat 4-6 healthy meals every day (behaviour goal). In three weeks, I want to have lost five pounds (outcome goal). As opposed to these short term goals, there are the long term goals. Ultimately, I want to weigh and maintain a weight of (fill in a suitable number based on information provided later in this chapter).

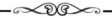

As you maintain new behaviours, you will be developing a new lifestyle for yourself, one that will undoubtedly translate into achieving your long term outcome goal.

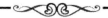

Download and use the Change4Good Goal Sheet© from **www.change4good.ca** to identify and track your long term goal, weekly (or short term) behaviour and outcomes goals, and strategies for achieving them. (Some behaviour goals, such as eat 4-6 nutritionally dense meals and/or snacks a day is a behaviour goal that is also a strategy). A sample of a completed Chang4Good Goal Sheet© is provided on page 44.

> **"The ultimate reason for setting goals is to entice you to become the person it takes to achieve them."**
> ~Jim Rohn, America's Foremost Business Philosopher
> *(Reprinted with permission from Jim Rohn International ©2011.)*

Goals can be unrealistic; they can be too grand and intimidating or too small and insignificant. To avoid either extreme, set reasonable goals.

The acronym *"Real Smart"* will help.

○ Ready for Obstacles

Be aware of potential obstacles so that you can develop strategies ahead of time. **Foresight allows you to take charge rather than react.**

○ Envision it

See yourself not only at your goal but on the road moving toward it. **Picture how you will look, feel and behave once you arrive; picture yourself taking the actions to get there** (tossing 2 ounces of almonds into a zip lock; saying 'no thank you').

○ Authentic

Your goal has to be yours, not what someone else wants for you. How many times in my practice do I see parents bringing in daughters, or a spouse bringing in their partner to lose weight? **If you don't want it, it won't happen.**

○ Live

Live as if you have already achieved your goal. **Eat, act, and dress as if you are who you hope to become.** Eat like a fit person; exercise like an athlete; dress for the job you want not the one you have. I have a friend who refused to buy new pants after she had gained a lot of weight. When she finally did buy a pair of pants that fit her properly, she felt better, and when you feel better, you're more inspired to make positive changes.

Specific

The more specific your goals, the better. **If you want to lose weight – specify how much. If you want to become more fit – identify what you want to be able to do.** "I want to lose ten pounds by my birthday." Or "I want to run 10km in 45 minutes." The smaller, short term goals will eventually yield the long term goal. Remember to maintain the previous week's goal as you start the new week's goal. If, after a week, you feel you haven't fully mastered the previous week's goal, stick with it until it – like Change4Good principles, becomes part of your life.

Measurable

Pick goals you can measure and then select a method for monitoring your progress. **You don't want to get hung up on numbers or mileposts but they do fix you in reality.** When they indicate progress, they're inspiring; when they don't, they enable you to reassess. **Monitoring keeps you from drifting off into that infamous state: denial.**

It may be as simple as monitoring:

- The number of pounds you lose each week.
- The number of centimetres you lose each month.
- The distance you can now walk or run.
- The number of the Change4Good Principles you are consistently incorporating on a daily basis.

Attainable

Your goals should be just grand enough to inspire you, but not so grand that they overwhelm you.

You may want to lose 15 pounds in a month, but losing at that rate may not be realistic or even desirable. On the other hand, sticking with 5-pound weights because you know you can lift them won't produce either the muscles you want or the energy that comes from pushing yourself that extra distance. **You may want to subject your goals to the reality test of running them by a knowledgeable professional.**

Recorded in Writing

Statistics show that people, who write down their goals, are significantly more likely to achieve them. **Writing not only keeps you honest; like prayer, it gives you one more minute in the day to remind you of your true destination.**

Time Sensitive

Deadlines save lives. They cause you to focus and commit. Also, they free you from the misery of procrastination. Again, chose a time frame that's realistic. You can't prepare to run a marathon in two weeks; on the other hand, taking two years is a sure way to deplete your enthusiasm. Again, once you've established your time frame, it may be wise to run it by a knowledgeable mentor or professional.

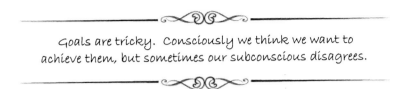

Goals are tricky. Consciously we think we want to achieve them, but sometimes our subconscious disagrees.

A good way to subject your goals to the 'do-I-really-want-this' **test**, is to consider what will happen when you achieve them. What will your life be like? **Ask yourself the following questions:**

- *How will I feel when I achieve my goal?* The status quo, however, undesirable, is, at least familiar. Some people are made to "pay" for getting healthy. A student who has always done poorly in school may lose his old gang if he decides to study harder or starts getting good grades.

  The classic case involves the woman who loses weight and suddenly finds herself eliciting unexpected male attention. **Sometimes, even the people who love us most, our spouses or our parents, are frightened by our changing.** And no one ever likes to lose an eating, drinking or moping buddy.

  The price you pay for not thinking through your goals or the consequences of achieving them is self-sabotage. I see it all the time: people lose significant amounts of weight and just as they approach their goal, they relapse. Why? As we said earlier, a new onslaught of attention, feelings, and even opportunities may frighten them. Unconsciously they may wish to return to their unhappy former self. At least s/he was familiar to them.

Just because achieving a certain goal may evoke uncomfortable feelings, however, doesn't mean you shouldn't pursue it. Rather, it reminds you to prepare for the problems you anticipate. Find new, supportive friends. Or discuss your plans with your spouse or loved ones so that they don't feel left out or frightened by your attempt, but included in it. They may even want to help.

Obstacles, considered at the beginning of a journey have less of a chance of subverting you. You have already anticipated them and taken steps to defuse them. Being ready is always preferable to being surprised.

Other questions to ask yourself:

- What resources do I need? Depending on your goals, a few sessions with a personal trainer or nutritionist might be in order; maybe cooking lessons; if your goal involves money, an hour or two with a financial planner might help.

- Will I be able to maintain my desired outcome? Just when you thought you had that work-out schedule nailed down, you receive an assignment that makes evening visits to the gym impossible. Deal creatively. Buy a treadmill for your home. A "no" answer to this question may also suggest that your goal is unwise. If your food plan is too restrictive or inflexible, it may not be able to accommodate to the real world. Losing too much weight too quickly also results in another, less obvious pitfall than muscle loss and stress; it may cause you to unnecessarily focus on food.

- *Do I know someone who has achieved a similar goal who can advise me?* When you find such people, use them. See what they do and ask how. Then return the favour to the universe by passing along the information you've received to another person it could help.

GUIDELINES FOR SETTING BODY COMPOSITION GOALS

Traditionally, the majority of clients working the Change4Good program want to achieve one very immediate goal: they want to lose weight. Let's first clarify a few things. First of all, when I talk about losing weight, I'm talking about losing body fat. Who cares if you lose three pounds but it's mostly water? Worse, what if it's muscle? It's healthier to be heavier and have more muscle and less body fat than to be thinner and have more body fat and less muscle. In other words, **numbers on a scale, although important, aren't the whole story.**

Therefore, you want to track all of the following:
- Body weight
- Waist-to-hip ratio or waist measurement
- Body fat percentage

The combination will give you an accurate benchmark of whether your body weight and composition are in the healthy range and at what rate it's changing.

Recently, I've been working with a client whose goal is to lose weight/body fat.

- At the three-month point, her measurements showed that she has lost about 13 pounds – approximately a pound a week – which meets the criteria of being consistent and healthy. She, on the other hand, was really hoping to have lost more at this point.
- Her measurements, however, told a more dramatic story. In three months, she had lost a total of 15.4 inches, which is remarkable.
- Also, the area of her body for which we did the most weight training was also the area that registered the greatest loss in terms of inches.

If we had just monitored her weight, her results would have seemed quite ordinary; taking into account her measurements, however, her results are far from average. The outcome underscores the importance of weight training in losing inches and changing body composition. She lost weight and fat and gained muscle; in other words, instead of being thin and flabby she's thin and buff. How cool is that? The moral of the story is: don't rely on weight alone.

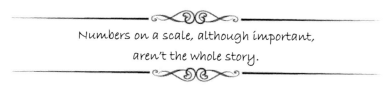

Numbers on a scale, although important,

aren't the whole story.

The charts on the following pages will give you some general guidelines for setting your body composition goals. **Remember, they're general.** Individual factors such as muscle mass, bone structure, age, body type and activity level must also be considered.

BODY WEIGHT

In terms body weight, here are some good rules of thumb:

What should your goal weight be?

WOMEN	MEN
100 lbs per 5 feet; add an additional 5 lbs per inch	106 lbs per 5 feet; add an additional 6 lbs per inch
Example: If you are 5'6", a good weight to aim for is 130lbs	Example: If you are 5'6", a good weight to aim for is 142lbs

What should you aim for in terms of weight loss per week?

The answer varies

Two pounds per week is too little for a person starting off at 250 pounds, and too much for a woman who merely wants to improve her ratio of lean muscle to fat mass.

Generally speaking, for the non-obese, a safe amount to lose in a week is 1-2 pounds. If you are losing much more, chances are it's water or muscle, or both, neither of which you want to lose.

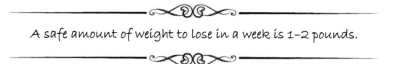

A safe amount of weight to lose in a week is 1-2 pounds.

A reasonable rate of body fat loss is about 1-2% per month. *(See healthy body fat ranges on page 42).* Be patient. Your body will adapt. It's your mind that may give you trouble. **Follow the 10 Change4Good Principles© consistently and the changes in your body composition will happen at exactly the right time.**

One more warning about weight: body fat, as we'll see, is harder to measure than pure weight. For this reason, people focus more on weight than body fat.

Remember, though, people are far more healthy and attractive when they weigh more and have less body fat than when they weigh less and have flab.

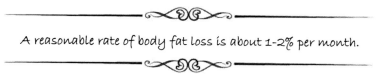

A reasonable rate of body fat loss is about 1-2% per month.

WAIST-TO-HIP RATIO MEASUREMENT

Waist-hip ratios (WHR) gauge body fat distribution. The latter is important as an indicator of the likelihood of developing certain types of disease. **Having excess body fat in the abdomen area, which is typical of an apple-shaped body type, creates the greatest risk for heart disease, diabetes, hypertension and other major ailments.** Storing more fat in your hip area, the classic pear shape, lowers your risk.

The following chart lists the guidelines for a healthy WHR:

WOMEN	MEN
Less than 0.8	Less than 1.0

To calculate your WHR:
- Take your waist measurement (measuring at the midpoint between the 12th rib and the top of the hip bone).
- Take your hip measurement (measuring at the widest point).
- Then divide your waist measurement (the smaller number) by your hip measurement (the larger number).

For example: If a woman's waist measures 25 inches and her hips measure 36 inches, her WHR is 0.69 which would place her in the healthy range for WHR.

Or, to make life easier, once you have your waist and hip measurements, use the body composition calculators at: **www.jawno.com/content/calculators/whr.shtml.**

WAIST ONLY MEASUREMENT

Alternatively, you could just keep track of your waist measurements. It, too, will indicate your risk of disease as a result of excess body fat in the abdomen area (although unlike WHR, it does not indicate comparatively where the excess fat is stored). Your waist measurement should be less than half of your height.

The following chart lists the guidelines for a healthy waist measurement:

WOMEN	MEN
Less than 35 in. or 89 cm	Less than 40 in. or 102 cm

BODY FAT

The most accurate way to measure your body fat is either **Dual-Energy X-Ray Absorptiometry (DXA)** or **hydrostatic (underwater) weighing.** Unfortunately both methods require expensive equipment that isn't widely available.

You could also find a professional who could measure skin fold thickness with an instrument called a calliper. The accuracy of these results, however, depends entirely on the experience and skill of the person taking the measurements.

Perhaps an easier method is one that uses **bioelectrical impedance analysis (BIA).** Both water and electrolytes conduct electricity. Body fat resists the flow of electricity because fat tissue contains less water and fewer electrolytes than lean tissue. Using a special device, a monitor sends a painless, low voltage electrical current through your body.

The device then converts information it receives on the body's electrical resistance into an estimate of total body fat. The accuracy of this measurement is contingent amongst other things, on the subject's level of hydration. In other words, the more dehydrated you are, the more distorted the reading. Bathroom scales and certain handheld devices also use this technology. The margin of error in these devices is too large for, say, elite athletes but for the rest of us, acceptable, providing a reasonable benchmark from which to work. (Professional devices using this technology tend to be more accurate than home versions such as bathroom scales).

If you know your height, weight, waist and hip measurements, you can find your approximate level of body fat at the body composition calculators at:
www.jawno.com/content/calculators/body-fat.shtml

The American Council on Exercise[5] gives the following guidelines for healthy body fat percentages for adult women and men:

WOMEN		MEN	
Essential	10 - 13%	Essential	2 – 5%
Athletes	14 – 20%	Athletes	6 – 13%
Fitness	21 – 24%	Fitness	14 – 17%
Acceptable	25 – 31%	Acceptable	18 – 24%
Obese	32% plus	Obese	25% plus

- **Essential:** refers to the amount of fat you need to be considered healthy. Women with less than 10-13 percent body fat may stop menstruating, for example. Among *athletes*, percentages vary. Swimmers need a higher percentage of body fat than, say, sprinters.

- **Fitness:** denotes a healthy ideal for the general population.

- **Acceptable:** means not ideal but, well, acceptable (you're probably slightly overweight).

- **Obese:** means you're at risk for major health problems.

Reminder: Again, numbers matter. You'll want to write them down on your **Change4Good Goal Sheet**© (see page 45) every week so that you know the results of your actions. In this manner you can't be in "denial". With the hundreds of clients I have worked with over the years, I have found that people who weigh themselves often (one to two times per week), and consistently are best at catching and losing new pounds before they become fat.

CHANGE4GOOD GOAL SHEET©

On the next page is a sample of a completed
Change4Good Goal Sheet©.

To download your Change4Good Goal Sheet© go to
www.change4good.ca.

Change Your Behaviours

Sample Change4Good Goal Sheet©

My Long Term Goal:			
Lose 25 pounds in 6 months starting December 1.			

My Short Term (Weekly) Goals:

DATE *December 1*			
Measurements	**Behaviour Goal**	**Strategy**	**Outcome Goal**
Weight *165 lbs* **Waist** *36 in* **Body Fat** *34%*	*Add a non starchy vegetable serving to every meal*	*Buy precut washed vegetables*	*Lose 1 lb at the end of this week; manage appetite*

DATE *December 8*	**How Did I Do?** *I added a vegetable serving at lunch and dinner but not breakfast* *Lost 1 lb*		**What I Will Change?** *Have a vegetable serving as one snack*
Measurements	**Behaviour Goal**	**Strategy**	**Outcome Goal**
Weight *164 lbs* **Waist** *36 in* **Body Fat** *34%*	*Increase water intake to three 500ml bottles per day*	*Keep a water bottle with me at all times*	*Lose 1 lb at the end of this week; manage appetite*

DATE *December 15*	**How Did I Do?** *I added a vegetable serving as one snack every day* *I drank three 500ml bottles per day* *Lost 1.5 lbs*		**What I Will Change?** *Increase to four 500ml bottles per day*
Measurements	**Behaviour Goal**	**Strategy**	**Outcome Goal**
Weight *162.5 lbs* **Waist** *36 in* **Body Fat** *34%*	*Have one protein shake with fruit each day*	*Keep blender on kitchen counter and buy frozen fruit*	*Lose 1 lb at the end of this week; manage appetite*

Change4Good Goal Sheet

My Long Term Goal:			

My Short Term (Weekly) Goals:			
DATE			
Measurements	Behaviour Goal	Strategy	Outcome Goal
Weight			
Waist			
Body Fat			
DATE	How Did I Do?		What I Will Change?
Measurements	Behaviour Goal	Strategy	Outcome Goal
Weight			
Waist			
Body Fat			
DATE	How Did I Do?		What I Will Change?
Measurements	Behaviour Goal	Strategy	Outcome Goal
Weight			
Waist			
Body Fat			

Goodies Department:

Reward yourself along the way at a point that seems reasonable as an additional incentive to stay on track. For example, when I lose 10 pounds, I'll buy a new pair of jeans, get a massage, get tickets for a concert or baseball game.

JOURNALING

Research shows that people who keep food journals have the greatest success at losing weight and maintaining their loss. One study, for example, conducted by Kaiser Permanente's Center for Health Research (which was also conducted at Duke University Medical Center and John Hopkins University), found that the more you track your food intake, the more weight you are likely to lose.

Why?

- Because writing down your mood, what you are eating, how much you are eating, even the weather, makes you aware and accountable of your immediate choices.
- Paying attention to your mood can specifically help reduce emotional eating.
- When you track the quantity of food you eat, you become very aware of portions. Without measuring and tracking food intake, most people underestimate calorie intake by 20–60%.
- Writing down what you **will** eat gives you time to pause and reflect upon the impact of your potential choice, on your goals and gives you the opportunity to maybe change that decision.[6]

Simply by recording what he'd eaten in his journal, a participant in one of my seminars called to tell me two weeks after he'd heard me speak, his weight dropped two pounds. Writing down what he ate made him aware of some of his less helpful patterns, like over-eating and unhealthy afternoon snacking, and adopt healthier ones, like eating smaller meals and not always running up for seconds.

In my own case, at one point, I thought I was eating chocolate a couple of times a week. Couple of times a week was, in fact, almost every day.

Another client said that keeping a journal revealed the awful truth: she was – literally – having a litre of lattes a day. She knew she drank a lot of lattes, but a litre? The lattes weren't a problem because of the calories they involved – she was an athlete eager to improve her performance, not count calories – but because of the nutrients she was losing by filling up on lattes.

About 30-40 percent of my clients are performance oriented. The poor eating habits of some of even the most talented among them astonishes me. The quality – not just the quantity – of what you eat affects your health and performance as well.

The Change4Good Journal© allows you to note other factors that might influence your eating.

"Why am I eating so much starchy stuff?" you may wonder. Maybe you're cold and tired of winter. Try soup. Mood is another factor. Do you feel bad because you hit the vending machines? Maybe you hit the vending machines because you were feeling bad. What produced those bad feelings? Is there a more effective way to deal with them? "If it wasn't for weekends, I'd be thin," a client told me the other day. Since weekends aren't going to end any time soon, she needs to know how to manage them: go to a movie instead of dinner, or do both, but pick a restaurant that serves foods that you adore and that are healthy. (Or, jump to the section on managing "treats" in Chapter EIGHT).

Unfortunately, some clients see having a bad day as an excuse to stop record-keeping. They can't bear to record the entire pizza they consumed, viewing the error as a blight on their soul or in their journal. Refrain. You're human. You're going to have bad days. If you continue to record them, however, they're more likely to decrease. Personally, nothing motivates me to get back on track more than reviewing a previous day's not-so-healthy entry.

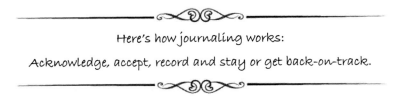

Here's how journaling works:

Acknowledge, accept, record and stay or get back-on-track.

This simple progression will keep things (i.e. your weight) from getting out of control.

For decades, I've kept my journal in a variety of spiral notebooks. The current one sits on my kitchen counter when I'm home; when I go out, I toss it into my bag. What about the inconvenience? Are you really going to carry your journal with you when all you're carrying is a small evening bag? A tennis racket? Your clubs? Not a problem. Write it on a piece of paper or send yourself a text message *(in situ)*; then write it in your journal when you get home. If you wait until you get home to record it, you'll probably leave something out.

Benefits of Journaling:

- Makes you think about what and why you are eating.

- Helps you become a more conscious and intentional eater.

- Keeps you aware of your food portions.

- Keeps you accountable to yourself.

- Helps identify patterns of eating.

- Helps motivate you to stay on track or get back on track.

- Can show you patterns between your energy, mood, the weather and your eating.

- Helps you monitor the extent to which you are following the 10 Change4Good Principles©.

To get you started, download your Change4Good Journal© at **www.change4good.ca.** If you're more high tech, download comparable applications to help you monitor yourself each day.

On the next few pages are two sample days from my personal food journal. These, together with the ones on pages 132-135 will not only show you how to complete the Change4Good Journal©, but will also give you ideas on how to apply Principles 4, 5 and 7 to your daily eating plan.

Change4Good Journal© – Sample #1

Date:	*April 5 2011*		LP: Lean Protein, NC: Natural Carbs, HF: Healthy Fats, O: Other	
Weather	☀ ☁ ☁	Energy Level ⬆ ➡ ⬇	Mood ☺ ☺ ☹	
Time	**Meal/Snack 1: What I Ate**			**Portion**
8:00 a.m	*Oatmeal with protein powder*			
	LP: *Protein powder (mixed into oatmeal)*			*1 scoop*
	NC: *Oatmeal*			*½ cup*
	HF: *Ground Flaxseed*			*1 tbsp*
	O: *Tea with 2% milk*			.
Weather	☀ ☁ ☁	Energy Level ⬆ ➡ ⬇	Mood ☺ ☺ ☹	
Time	**Meal/Snack 2: What I Ate**			**Portion**
10:45 a.m	*Apple and raw almonds*			
	LP:			
	NC: *Apple*			*1 med*
	HF: *Raw almonds*			*10*
	O:			
Weather	☀ ☁ ☁	Energy Level ⬆ ➡ ⬇	Mood ☺ ☺ ☹	
Time	**Meal/Snack 3: What I Ate**			**Portion**
1:30 pm	*Tuna sandwich with vegetables*			
	LP: *Tuna*			*1 can*
	NC: *Spelt bread, peppers and carrots*			*2 slices, ¼ cup*
	HF:			
	O: *Salsa*			*2 tbsp*
Water	▨ ▨ ▨ ▨ ▨ ▨ ▨ ▨ ▨ ▨ ☐ ☐			
Supplements	*Omega – 3, Juice Plus, Vitamin D3, Maca Powder*			

Change4Good Journal© – Sample #1

LP: Lean Protein, NC: Natural Carbs, HF: Healthy Fats, O: Other

Weather ☀ ⛅ (🌧)	Energy Level ↑ (↔) ↓	Mood (☺) ☺ ☹
Time	**Meal/Snack 4: What I Ate**	**Portion**
4:15 pm	Banana and cheese	
	LP: Babybel light cheese	1
	NC: Banana	1 small
	HF:	
	O:	

Weather ☀ (⛅) 🌧	Energy Level ↑ (↔) ↓	Mood (☺) ☺ ☹
Time	**Meal/Snack 5: What I Ate**	**Portion**
7:30 pm	Beef stir fry with Shirataki noodles	
	LP: Lean beef	3 oz
	NC: Shirataki noodles, frozen vegetables	1 packet, ¾ cup
	HF: Olive oil in pasta sauce	
	O: Pasta sauce	½ cup

Weather ☀ (⛅) (🌧)	Energy Level ↑ (↔) ↓	Mood (☺) ☺ ☹
Time	**Meal/Snack 6: What I Ate**	**Portion**
10:00 pm	Stewed apples with yogurt	
	LP: Greek yogurt	2 tbsp
	NC: Stewed apples	¾ cup
	HF:	
	O:	

Workout Summary	Cardio – 30 minute run (5pm)

Change4Good Journal© – Sample #2

Date: *April 10 2011*		LP: Lean Protein, NC: Natural Carbs, HF: Healthy Fats, O: Other

Weather ☀ ☁ 🌧	Energy Level ↑ → ↓	Mood 😊 😐 ☹

Time	Meal/Snack 1: What I Ate	Portion
9:30 am	Protein Pancake	
	LP: *Egg whites*	*½ cup*
	NC: *Uncooked oatmeal, unpasteurized honey*	*¼ cup, 2 tsp*
	HF: *Ground Flaxseed*	*2 tbsp*
	O: *Tea with 2% milk*	

Weather ☀ ☁ 🌧	Energy Level ↑ → ↓	Mood 😊 😐 ☹

Time	Meal/Snack 2: What I Ate	Portion
12:30 pm	Veggie burger and 4 bean salad	
	LP: *Veggie burger*	*1 Patti*
	NC: *Bean salad, steamed frozen vegetables*	*½ cup, 1 cup*
	HF: *Salad dressing with olive oil*	*1 tbsp*
	O:	

Weather ☀ ☁ 🌧	Energy Level ↑ → ↓	Mood 😊 😐 ☹

Time	Meal/Snack 3: What I Ate	Portion
3:45 pm	Elevate Me Bar	*1 bar*
	LP: *Elevate Me Bar*	
	NC: *Elevate Me Bar*	
	HF:	
	O: *Tea with 2% milk*	

Water	🥛🥛🥛🥛🥛🥛🥛🥛🥛🥛🥛🥛
Supplements	*Omega – 3, Juice Plus, Vitamin D3, Maca Powder*

Change4Good Journal© – Sample #2

				LP: Lean Protein, NC: Natural Carbs, HF: Healthy Fats, O: Other			

Weather ☀ ⛅ ☁	Energy Level ↑ ↔ ↓	Mood ☺ 😐 ☹
Time	**Meal/Snack 4: What I Ate**	**Portion**
7:00 pm	Scrambled eggs and toast	
	LP: Eggs	2
	NC: Rice bread, grilled tomatoes onion and mushrooms	2 slices, ½ cup
	HF: Butter	1 tsp
	O:	

Weather ☀ ⛅ ☁	Energy Level ↑ ↔ ↓	Mood ☺ 😐 ☹
Time	**Meal/Snack 5: What I Ate**	**Portion**
10:15 pm	Banana and almond butter	
	LP:	
	NC: Banana	1 med
	HF: Almond butter	1 tsp
	O:	

Weather ☀ ⛅ ☁	Energy Level ↑ ↔ ↓	Mood ☺ 😐 ☹
Time	**Meal/Snack 6: What I Ate**	**Portion**
	LP:	
	NC:	
	HF:	
	O:	

Workout Summary	Weights – 45 minutes – full body (5:30pm)

Change Your Behaviours

Change4Good Journal©

Date:						LP: Lean Protein, NC: Natural Carbs, HF: Healthy Fats, O: Other		
Weather	☀	⛅	🌧	Energy Level	↑ ↔ ↓	Mood	☺ ☻ ☹	
Time	Meal/Snack 1: What I Ate					Portion		
	LP							
	NC							
	HF							
	O							
Weather	☀	⛅	🌧	Energy Level	↑ ↔ ↓	Mood	☺ ☻ ☹	
Time	Meal/Snack 2: What I Ate					Portion		
	LP							
	NC							
	HF							
	O							
Weather	☀	⛅	🌧	Energy Level	↑ ↔ ↓	Mood	☺ ☻ ☹	
Time	Meal/Snack 3: What I Ate					Portion		
	LP							
	NC							
	HF							
	O							
Water	🥛 🥛 🥛 🥛 🥛 🥛 🥛 🥛 🥛 🥛							
Supplements								

Change4Good Journal©

LP: Lean Protein, NC: Natural Carbs, HF: Healthy Fats, O: Other		
Weather ☀ ☁ ☔	Energy Level ↑ ↔ ↓	Mood ☺ ☺ ☹
Time	Meal/Snack 4: What I Ate	Portion
	LP	
	NC	
	HF	
	O	
Weather ☀ ☁ ☔	Energy Level ↑ ↔ ↓	Mood ☺ ☺ ☹
Time	Meal/Snack 5: What I Ate	Portion
	LP	
	NC	
	HF	
	O	
Weather ☀ ☁ ☔	Energy Level ↑ ↔ ↓	Mood ☺ ☺ ☹
Time	Meal/Snack 6: What I Ate	Portion
	LP	
	NC	
	HF	
	O	
Workout Summary		

Some additional tips to ensure successful journaling include:

- If you use something other than the Change4Good Journal© provided, make sure you are tracking all the same components as outlined in the Change4Good Journal©: time of meals, contents, portions, how much water (or other beverages) you drink, supplements taken; exercise performed; energy level, mood – even the weather if it's relevant.

- Keep the journal with you whenever possible, as you would a driver's license or a good-luck object.

- Write down what you eat or drink immediately before – or after you have it. Some people prefer to write down what they plan to eat before they eat it. It helps them stay on track, especially on days that are emotionally or physically more challenging.

- Review your journal every couple of days or at the end of the week. Identify the patterns you want to reinforce. Analyze the ones you want to change and perhaps the cause of them. Strategize improvements. Regarding this principle and all others, **strive for moderation and consistency, not perfection.**

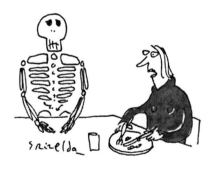

Srixella

www.cartoonstock.com

'I TOLD YOU NOT TO GO ON A
NO CARB , NO FAT , NO MEAT DIET
ALL AT ONCE...'

CHANGE4GOOD – ACTION STEPS

- Start implementing Principle 2 – Set Goals; Keep a Journal.

- Identify your Long Term Goal: For example: Lose 25 pounds in six months; lose 5% body fat in six months; train for a 10km run in 10 weeks; within 2 months be eating vegetarian 2 days per week.

- Identify and complete your first Short Term (weekly) Goal: For example: Buy a tape measure to track measurements; hire a personal trainer; register for a 5km run; cleanse self-talk e.g., "I am getting fitter with every step I take" instead of "I'm so out of shape."

- Update Change4Good Journal© daily.

- Update Change4Good Goal Sheet© weekly.

TOOLS

- Change4Good Goal Sheet©

- Change4Good Journal©

REMEMBER THIS

- People who write down what they eat on a daily basis generally lose more weight. **It's that simple.**

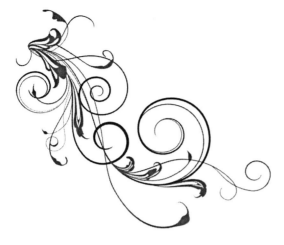

OBSTACLE COURSE: LIFE LESSONS

This chapter is about identifying the blocks that derail you, and moving around, over or through them.

Principle **3** Identify Barriers; *Surmount Them*

It's an un-vicious circle: the more sanely you live, the more sanely you'll eat. This chapter helps you identify your demons and vanquish them.

> **"The greatest glory in living lies not in never failing but in rising every time we fall."**
> ~Nelson Mandela, President of South Africa (1994 – 1999)

Instead of thrusting a food and exercise plan at you (and admit it: some of you want this), I'm going to spend some time here preparing you for all those bumps in the road you know you're going to hit. And good: hit them. Life is not about things going smoothly; it's about hanging in there when they don't. That's when you grow muscles – both in your body and in your character. Over the years, I've observed hundreds of clients confront numerous barriers in their drive to live and eat healthily. The key to succeeding in almost every case was for them to **change their behaviour.** Below are 15 of the most common barriers that sabotage even the best of intentions.

Changing your attitude was covered in detail in Chapter ONE (Principle 1).

The following four will be covered in subsequent chapters:

- Infrequent and poor quality meals/snacks (Solution: Chapter FOUR and FIVE, Principle 4 and 5).
- Lack of nutritional planning and preparation (Solution: Chapter SIX and SEVEN, Principle 6).
- Poor portion management (Solution: Chapter SEVEN, Principle 7).
- Lack of moderation when eating out (Solution: Chapter EIGHT, Principle 8).

In this chapter, the following 10 behaviours and the barriers they fuel will be addressed. They are:

Behaviour	Barrier
1: Disorganized	1: Time Deprived
2: Inadequate Stress Management	2: Lack of Energy and Stamina
3: Poor Sleep Habits	3: Sleep Deprived
4: Emotional Detachment	4: Eating to Escape
5: Relationship Dysfunction	5: Eating to Please/Escape
6: Perfectionism	6: All or Nothing Attitude
7: Nutritionally Unbalanced Diet	7: Cravings
8: Clean Plate Syndrome	8: Eat It Because It's There
9: Eat It Because Its Free (food samples, business events, airline lounges)	9: Unable to Stay on Track
10: Frozen	10: Stop Journaling, Stop Exercising

Change4Good Behaviour GPS©

Just as you did with the Attitude GPS©, you may want to construct a Behaviour GPS© just to help you pinpoint which of your current behaviours are fueling your largest barriers to healthy living. Note that in *this* GPS, the **less** a particular behaviour is an issue for you (in other words you disagree with it), the **lower the rating** you would give it; the **more** a behaviour is an issue for you (in other words you agree with it), the **higher the rating** you would give it. For example, if being disorganized (Behaviour 1) is not really an issue for you (you strongly disagree) then give it a score of 2. But if always eating food because it is free (Behaviour 9) is an issue for you (you strongly agree), give it a score of 10 for example, and so on.

Below is an example of a completed Change4Good Behaviour GPS©

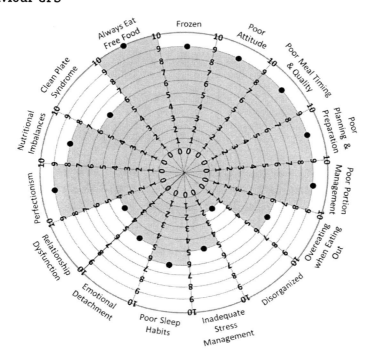

Your Change4Good Behaviour GPS©

For your own purposes use either the blank one on this page or download it at **www.change4good.ca.**

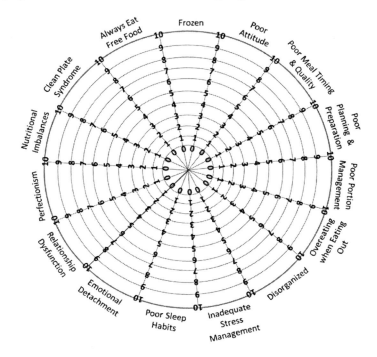

What to do:

1. Using the Change4Good Behaviour GPS© rate your level of **agreement/disagreement** for each separate area between zero and ten (**ten being complete agreement; zero being complete disagreement**).

2. Place one dot (per segment) opposite the number that best represents your level of agreement/disagreement.

3. Connect the dots to create a "circle" within the Change4Good Behaviour GPS©. **Unless you have no destructive behaviours or all are equally disturbing, the** circle-within-the-circle is bound to be *asymmetrical*.

Now, consider the following, remembering that this GPS is interpreted slightly differently from the others:

1. **How large is your circle?** Smaller is better.

2. **How symmetrical is it?** Your goal is to push everything to the center, to have the smallest, roundest circle.

3. **Where does your circle extend toward the outer rim? In this GPS, these are the areas that need the most attention.** You'll refer back to all 15 when you tackle the exercise at the end of this chapter. In the meantime, here are some suggestions for pushing each mini-arc inward.

SOLUTIONS TO OVERCOME COMMON DESTRUCTIVE BEHAVIOURS

You've diagnosed the problem; now let's get on with the solutions:

Disorganized

BARRIER: Poor Time Management

SOLUTION: Get Time Savvy

One of the greatest challenges my clients face is their perceived lack of time – to shop, cook, and exercise and even just live consciously. The day just seems to slip through their fingers.

How do they change that? They consciously monitor their time, and then become more organized and savvy with how to spend it.

An easy way to do that is via the **Change4Good Time Journal**© on the next page. Try it. If, in a few days, you decide that you prefer staring into space or watching television into the wee hours, you can always revert back to your old behaviour.

To begin: **Keep a diary of everything you do for a couple of days in the Change4Good Time Journal© ** (see example). Just as keeping a food journal did, keeping a Time Journal may also yield surprises: a whole day on the internet? A half day chatting with friends or watching TV? No wonder you didn't have time for that spin class, or weeding you wanted to do.

Sample Change4Good Time Journal© – Date: December 1

Date			
Time	Activity	Duration	Importance High/Medium/Low
6 50	Woke up	10 min	High
7 00	Showered; ready for work	30 min	High
7 30	Breakfast	20 min	High
7 50	Commuted to work	45 min	High
8 30	Lectured	3 hours	High
11 30	Lunch, checked emails	60 min	High
12 30	Lectured	3 hours	High
3 30	Responded to emails	1 hour	High
4 30	Commuted home	60 min	High
5 30	Checked emails; watched TV	60 min	Medium
6 30	Dinner	30 min	High
7	Personal Calls; watched TV	2 hours	Medium
9	Made lunch for next day	30 min	High
9 30	Watched TV; read	90 min	Low
11	Went to sleep		

	Activity	Duration	Possible Changes
SUMMARY	Travel	1 hr 45 min	
	Work	8 hrs	
	Meals - Preparation	30 min	
	Meals - Eating	1 hr	
	Phone Calls	1 – 1.5 hrs	Reduce to 45 min; use extra time to read or socialize
	Emails	1 hr	
	Television	3 hrs	Reduce to 1 hr.; use time to workout
	Social Activities		
	Working Out		
	Internet		
	Personal Hygiene	45 min	
	Hobbies/Recreation		

Identify Barriers; Surmount Them

Track how you are spending your time; use the Change4Good Time Journal© below or download one at **www.change4good.ca.**

Date			
Time	Activity	Duration	Importance High/Medium/Low

	Activity	Duration	Possible Changes
SUMMARY	Travel		
	Work		
	Meals - Preparation		
	Meals - Eating		
	Phone Calls		
	Emails		
	Television		
	Social Activities		
	Working Out		
	Internet		
	Personal Hygiene		
	Hobbies/Recreation		

Below are some strategies that may help you streamline and organize your life so that there is time for exercise and even just plain time (*time for time*)! In my own happily busy but sometimes overwhelming life, I use strategies 1, 2, and 3 daily, and a healthy dose of 5 and 6 throughout the week.

Review the list and see what you like. Yes, there are only 24 hours in a day, but using them wisely, it's amazing how rich and satisfying they can be.

1. **Buy/download and use a diary/organizer.**

   Write down your plans in whatever tool you choose: a Day-Timer©, iPhone©, Blackberry© or other application or software program.

2. **Prioritize.**

   At night or first thing in the morning, scan your "to do" list. Start with what absolutely has to get done. If you have 10 chores – a heavy load – postpone the three or four that can easily be done another day, and use that "freed up" time to shop for vegetables, prepare a batch of meals or maybe even tend your garden, meditate or do a favour for someone. It doesn't all have to be a rat race.

3. **Set boundaries.**

   Cede to requests, but carefully. Yes, you want to be a good daughter / son / parent / sibling / colleague / boss but you also need to say 'no' occasionally (or frequently) – to others and to yourself. For example, I don't even look at my emails before I work out in the morning. If I did, I'd never get to the gym. As a result, I've made it non-negotiable: workout first, then emails. When I do let myself take on certain chores, like emailing, I set a time limit. Otherwise, these activities can bleed into escapes.

Identify Barriers; Surmount Them

4. **Delegate.**

   Consider what you can pass on to someone else. Maybe involve your kids in meal preparation such as setting the table or chopping vegetables (they might even start to like baby carrots, tomatoes or sugar snap peas).

5. **Be productive while waiting.**

   Everyone has downtime (waiting for clients, responses, the hairdresser, the dentist). Some downtime is good, even recommended and necessary; but if you find yourself unable to accomplish your priority tasks – economize.

   Technology makes it easy. If I'm waiting for the hairdresser, out comes my laptop. I peck away at the article due that evening or update a client's program. Addicted to television news? Watch it while running on a treadmill.

6. **Limit distractions.**

   Block out time for the portion of your work that requires total concentration. Shut the door, turn off your phone and pager, and ignore the outer world. You won't die and either will it disappear. When I write, I ignore all distractions. When I don't, it takes me forever to reconnect to whatever train of thought I've lost. Better not to lose the connection in the first place. Remember our discussion on "un-multi task" in Chapter ONE?

7. **Know your work rhythms.**

   If you are a night person, don't schedule the heavy duty lifting (whether physical or mental) in the morning. Save those chores or problems for when your engines are up and running.

"It's not enough to be busy, so are the ants.
The question is: what are we busy about?"
~Henry David Thoreau, American Writer, Philosopher

Inadequate Stress Management

BARRIER: Lack of Energy and Stamina

SOLUTION: Bust Stress

Finally – you have that hour or so each day you need to exercise. Unfortunately, by the time you get home, you're too exhausted. Down you sink into the couch. Clearly, if you're exhausted long before bedtime, the energy doctor is required.

For starters, physical energy will improve by: eating wisely, exercising, staying hydrated, and getting quality sleep. It will also improve by acquiring better attitudes (see Chapter ONE). But another key aspect to managing energy is **managing stress** – physical, emotional, mental and even spiritual.

Eating well and exercising alleviates some stress but stress often causes us to eat poorly and bag out on exercise. The point being: it's important to manage stress so that it doesn't derail our other attempts to live a healthy life. Stress, therefore, needs to be managed – like food, like cravings, like rowdy children.

Try the obvious: some kind of restorative physical or mental activity. When I'm stressed out, going for a run works wonders: I physically, mentally and emotionally recharge and in the solitude of my running, work through problems that I couldn't previously untangle.

Sometimes talking to a good friend, meditating or writing in a diary or journal does it. The key is to recognize that stress is a silent killer – like a vampire, it sucks energy -- and arm yourself against it just as you do (and will after internalizing these principles) mindless eating.

For technocrats, here's a toy: the Desktop emWave®, a hardware and software program that, helps you monitor your heart rate variability (the coherence between your sympathetic nervous system/stress response and parasympathetic nervous system/relaxation response) via biofeedback as you focus on deep breathing and maybe even positive visualizations which can help set your mind, heart and emotions in a more balanced state and increase your overall capacity for what you have to deal with.

Poor Sleep Habits

> BARRIER: Sleep Deprived
>
> SOLUTION: Implement Sleep Strategies

Adults need approximately 8-8.5 hours of sleep. Some people do all right with as little as 5 hours; some swear they need 10. Regardless, you'll do better with at least 7-8 hours of quality sleep.

Sleep affects: mood, immune function, cardiovascular health, ability to learn and stay safe, memory, metabolism and weight. The effect of sleep deprivation on metabolism is related in part to altered hormone function.

Chronic sleep deprivation alters the level of two hormones, ghrelin and leptin. The gastrointestinal tract produces ghrelin, which stimulates appetite; fat cells produce leptin, which signals the brain when you are full.

When you are sleep deprived, your leptin levels decrease, which means you don't feel as satisfied as usual after a meal. Your ghrelin levels increase, which stimulates appetite and increases your desire for more food. The resulting fatigue also precipitates overeating. Tired, you're more likely to reach for food—bad food, fast food.

Ah, if only it were that simple. You probably yearn for more sleep but either don't have the time or the ability to rest those hours.

Comb the following strategies, to see which of them might help:

- Our sleep-wake cycle is regulated by what's known as a "circadian clock," an endogenous (built-in) mechanism that controls our biological rhythms. Although regulated internally, these rhythms respond to certain external cues. In terms of sleep, daylight is the most powerful. We sleep most easily when it's dark and wake up when it's light. **Keeping a regular sleep/wake schedule – that is, going to bed at say 11 p.m. and waking at 7:30 a.m. - even on weekends – helps guard against insomnia.**

- **If you wake up at night, don't look at your clock or better yet, put it away altogether.** According to experts, seeing the time when you wake in the middle of the night subconsciously trains your body to keep waking at that time. If you can, don't use an alarm clock. Go to sleep at an hour that will assure you're rising at the right time – naturally.

- **Don't consume stimulants – the obvious one is caffeine – within 4-6 hours of your bedtime.** Also limit your caffeine consumption in general. Caffeine remains in the body on average from 3-5 hours, but can affect some people up to 12 hours after consumption. Even if you don't think caffeine affects you – "I can drink coffee after dinner and go right to sleep," is a regular comment I hear, but it may be lessening the quality of your sleep in general.

- Nicotine is another stimulant. **Avoid smoking altogether but especially before bedtime.** Then again, smoking is a lose-lose proposition. Not smoking before bedtime causes your body to wake up prematurely on account of nicotine withdrawal. **Best solution: don't smoke, but then you already know that.**

- **Alcohol also disrupts sleep.** It may seem to lull you to sleep but it also disrupts it.

- **Avoid heavy meals and spicy foods close to bedtime; both can lead to discomfort during the night.** It is best not to eat within 2-3 hours of going to bed; limit liquid consumption as well to prevent pre-dawn trips to the bathroom.

- **Regular exercise is great but not too close to bedtime.** It is best to complete it a few hours before your bedtime. Exercise generally stimulates the body and raises body temperature – which detracts from sleep quality.

- **Avoid stimulating or stressful activities before bedtime: working, paying bills, engaging in emotional or upsetting conversations** (if you can help it). Instead, establish a regular and relaxing routine: a warm bath with lavender, a good book or soothing music – any activity that eases the transition into sleep.

> *"Man should forget his anger before he lies down to sleep."*
> ~Mahatma Gandhi

- **Check your mattress and pillows.** Mattresses should be replaced every 9-10 years and pillows, as soon as they look limp.

- **Restrict your bedroom for sleep or sleep-related activities** (i.e. sex). You want to reinforce the association between "bed" and "sleep." Remove from the bedroom computers or any item that creates anxiety.

- Light, as we said, directly affects the circadian sleep rhythm by stimulating the neurons that cause us to awaken. **Avoid bright light at night; also noise. The ideal sleep environment is cool, dark, quiet and comfortable.**

Emotional Detachment

> BARRIER: Eating to Escape (Emotional Eating)
>
> SOLUTION: Separate Food and Emotions

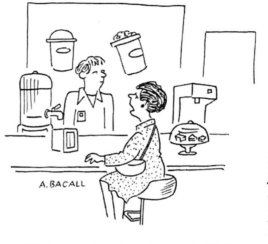

"It's been a rough day. Supersize my mocha latte."

www.cartoonstock.com

Emotional or stress eating is when you eat for reasons other than physical hunger – or pleasure up to a point.

The critical question is how do you know?

Spot check: Take a moment and ask yourself: how am I feeling? Angry? Depressed? Weary? Anxious? Euphoric?

Then travel back in time and try to figure out exactly what moment produced those feelings. Did you have a fight with someone earlier? Did you suffer a disappointment? Are you anxious about something; perhaps just the opposite, you're excited, elated, overjoyed. Scared?

Sometimes just knowing how you are feeling helps your body and mind adjust. Oh, so I'm angry. I'm not hungry. What should I do about that? Well sure you could eat but then you'd have two problems: anger and excess calories.

It's better to focus on what's really bothering you. Talk to a friend. Write in your journal. Meditate. Think. Run.

Give your mind a chance to process the flood of new feelings. Then you'll be better able to distinguish fake hunger from real. **The whole point of being conscious is to be thoughtful and aware rather than to mindlessly react.** When you handle your emotional problems honestly and well, you'll probably feel a state of happiness in which only real hunger survives.

"If you try to get rid of fear and anger without knowing
their meaning, they will grow stronger and return."

~Deepak Chopra

Additional strategies to help when emotions overwhelm:

- **Recognize and prepare for "trigger situations" as much as possible.** Dinner with the in-laws? Bathing suit shopping? Painful anniversary (or lack of one)? **The first step in handling these situations is to acknowledge them.** Then rehearse, visualize, analyze, discuss with a supportive friend. Call a friend before and after (and perhaps even during) the incident just to keep you sane.

- **Think before you eat;** this is where your journaling can be really helpful. Are you about to eat because you are physically hungry or because you are distressed? With practice, you'll learn to distinguish between real and emotional hunger. Knowing which you're feeling is half the battle.

- **Think about how you will feel afterwards.** Ask yourself: will what you are about to imbibe seem worth it tomorrow?

- **If it is too hard to truly confront the situation/your feelings at the time, distract yourself.** Grab your iPod. Take a walk. Play solitaire on the computer. Just remember that the sooner you deal with your feelings/the situation, the better.

- **Drink water or herbal tea** – the process, however simple, gives you time to think about what's really upsetting you. Certain herbal teas like camomile may actually help calm you.

- **Avoid having emotional conversations when you eat**, or eating when you are experiencing any extreme emotion whether it is anger, frustration, or anxiety.

- **Do what works for your personality.** Sing. Listen to music. I tidy and organize cupboards in my condo. Whether it's the physical activity of unpacking/folding/repacking – venting all my anger -- or simply the realization that I'm getting out of my own way -- it works. You feel better and in my case, I have cleaner cabinets too boot! **Gratitude** also helps. From A to Z, list 26 things in your life for which you're grateful. See if you don't feel just a little less surly.

"In the middle of difficulty lies opportunity."
~Albert Einstein, Physicist and Philosopher

Relationship Dysfunction

> BARRIER: Eating to Please (Emotional Eating)
>
> Eating to Escape (Emotional Eating)
>
> SOLUTION: Set Boundaries between Self and Others

Even some of our closest friends and family members, as well as some not so close, fear losing us when we change. Some eating or complaining-buddies will be loath to lose you as part of their crew. Let them see that the positive changes that you make will only make you a better roommate, spouse, lover or friend.

More specific to eating, some acquaintances fear you'll spoil the party if you don't join in. As time passes, you'll see – and they will too – that just because you aren't eating or drinking huge amounts, you can still relate, connect and share the good times.

Make sure you:

- **Separate your goals from those people around you when necessary.** Friendships worth keeping won't break over differences; they'll bend. Be prepared, however, for those friendships that may in fact break. We change. Our friends and acquaintances do too. It's not always a bad thing. Sometimes it's a sign of growth. Also, give your friends and loved ones time to adjust. As you grow, they may too.
- **Get support.** Cultivate a network of people/friends/family who can support you as you live with health and sanity.
- **Arrange social events that do not always revolve around food.** As hard this may sound, in time, it will seem as natural as food-dominated events once did. Remember moderation. You don't need to switch to bread and water; just de-emphasize the binge aspect.

Perfectionism

> BARRIER: *All-or-Nothing Attitude*
>
> SOLUTION: *Manage Those All-or-Nothing Attitudes*
>
> *Confront Rather Than Procrastinate*

How many times have you said, "I will get back on track tomorrow (or Monday or next month or after the holidays)?" Or, "well, I ate three cookies I might as well finish the box?" Or "I missed two workouts this week so I may as well blow the week and start again Monday?"

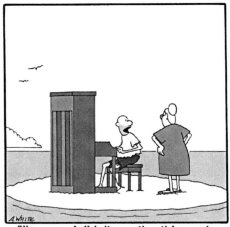

"I'm sorry I didn't practice this week,
Mrs. Tinklemeyer. I just had so
many distractions!"

It's not the three cookies or the two missed workouts that are going to set you back. It's the all or nothing attitude that will lead you to consume the whole box or miss the whole week, month or year.

Remember, consistency and moderation – not perfection.
You'll read more about this in Chapter EIGHT and Principle 8 (Practice: Moderation; Follow the 90/10 Rule).

In the meantime, perfectionism breeds fear and fear breeds procrastination. Avoid both. Do the best job you can. If you veer off track, don't plunge into the abyss.

Regarding food and fitness specifically:

If you have a bad meal, do not blow the whole day. Simply get back on track at the next snack or meal and consider these additional strategies:

1. Eat light at the next meal.
2. Make your next meal a protein and greens meal only.
3. Make your next meal a vegetable meal only.
4. Exercise that day.
5. If you had a complete day of unhealthy eating, follow either strategy number 2 or 3 for the entire next day.

> **"Every new beginning comes from some other beginning's end."**
> ~Seneca, Roman Philosopher

Nutritional Imbalances

     BARRIER: Cravings

     SOLUTION: Vanquish with Nutritionally Rich Meals

Chapter FIVE and Principle 5 relate to the dictum: Eat 4-6 nutrient dense meals/snacks per day. In the meantime, bear in mind the following:

- **Most North Americans are overfed and undernourished due to the poor quality of their diet.**
- **Our bodies cannot function optimally on chemicals, sugar, artificial flavours, and fast foods.**

- **Our bodies crave what we give them most;** subsist on sugar and processed food and that's what you'll crave. At the same time, you'll be hungry for the foods your body needs: protein, fat, carbohydrates, vitamins, minerals, and water -- in other words, real food. **Eat real food and eventually, junk will lose 99% of its appeal.**

The best way to eliminate cravings is to implement the 10 Change4Good Principles© laid out in this book.

Along the way, here are tips that will help:

- **Break the Sugar Cycle (real or artificial).** Some researchers maintain that just the taste of sugar creates a yearning for sweet food.

Artificial sweeteners have been shown to increase sugar cravings and appetite due to their effect on both blood sugar and serotonin levels.

For example, when we consume something sweet, like diet pop, the sweet taste stimulates the tongue and brain. The body is then conditioned to expect the arrival of new energy. Then you drink your can of diet pop but the body gets no energy. To compensate, the body produces signals that urge you to eat sugar. In general, this urge can last for up to 90 minutes. The moral of the story; **avoid fake – and real – sweeteners as a rule.**

- **Downsize Desire.** Often a mere 100 calories or spoonful of the craved item will do. Almost everything is available in a mini version.

- **Dental Defense.** Brush your teeth for a full minute and then meticulously floss them. Still want that chocolate? Didn't think so. If you cannot brush your teeth, suck on a mint. Makes you want to keep that clean feeling.

- **Dilute Sugar's Impact.** Add protein or a healthy fat to your carbohydrate meal. Put nut butter on your apple; toss chicken onto your pasta. Your blood sugar levels will remain more stable and your cravings will lessen in intensity.

- **Change the Habit** – if you are accustomed to having chocolate every afternoon at 3pm, try an all-natural health bar. Or have only two squares of the chocolate. Note: some people can handle only 2 squares of chocolate. Personally, I can't. I'd rather have an apple and cheese and save the chocolate bar for when I can eat all of it. Therefore, I save chocolate for my 90/10 treat. Which is to say: any rule is meant to be tweaked to your personal style.

- **Practice Mind Over Matter.** Our brains respond to visual images. Just seeing an image of pizza for example, can lead to cravings for pizza. To avoid these urges, bleep out the commercials on television or use that time to do a chore or even better some push-ups or squats. When an urge does strike, people have been known to use any number of tools: count backwards, phone a friend – before you know it, the craving will be gone. **The best way to eliminate cravings is not to feed them.**

- **Bite it, Chew it, Suck it.** Mood affects texture. When we are angry, we tend to crave something into which we can bite. I had a friend who binged on M&M's monthly after frustrating condominium board meetings. Switching to pretzels helped some; switching to carrots helped more. When upset, some people tend to crave something soothing and warm. Try vanilla herbal tea instead of a latte; oatmeal with cinnamon instead of apple pie.

- **Eat 4–6 Nutrient Dense Meals/Snacks throughout the day** to avoid blood sugar levels crashing (See Chapter FIVE, Principle 5).

Clean Plate Syndrome

   BARRIER: *Eat It Cause It's There*

   SOLUTION: *Vanquish with Nutritionally Rich Meals*

Did your parents instil in you the belief that it was shameful to waste food? It may be in many circumstances, but there are better ways of dealing with excess food than eating it:

- **Decide ahead of time how much food you will eat** – ½ of what is on your plate, ¾ of what is on your plate – and immediately put the rest aside or wrap it up to take for your lunch the next day.

- **Use a smaller plate** (see Chapter SEVEN on cool, reduced-size tableware).

- **When dining out, share a main course or order an appetizer as a main course with a salad.**

Eat it Cause it's Free

> BARRIER: Unable to Stay on Track
>
> SOLUTION: Develop New Strategies

Do you feel the need to eat free food because it's free? Hors d'oeuvres in an airline lounge while travelling? Samples while shopping? A food gift from someone? Strategies to help you cope with free food: Chew gum, sip water, say "No".

See if you identify with the following situation:

- A favourite aunt offers you a slice of her famous just-baked cheesecake. What do you say? "Oh, that looks beautiful. How I wish I could have a piece. Unfortunately, my stomach is a bit upset. I would adore it if you would give me a piece to take home and enjoy later."

- Every workshop at a business meeting is accompanied by a surfeit of treats; social events as well. Skip the pastries and head for the fruit and cheese platter. Or make those important connections while everyone else is eating. You might actually enjoy these events better with only a glass of sparkling water in your hand; keeps you clear-headed and alert. You snicker? Try it.

Recently, I went out for dinner with a colleague. Unfortunately, the service was slow and our order was not correct. To make amends, the manager sent out a complimentary dessert at the end of the meal. I didn't want to eat the dessert and neither did my colleague but we also didn't want to appear ungrateful. What did we do? We offered it to the couple at the next table. In the end, everyone went home happy.

Memorize these responses:

- *"Oh thank you so much. That looks wonderful. Unfortunately, I just had a big meal and couldn't possibly manage another bite (even though of course you could – but won't)."*

- *"I'd love to but I have a big dinner coming up tonight. Another time?"*

- *"I'm sorry but I don't eat blank (cake, cookies, white sugar, flour...)" or "I'm allergic to (this, that and the other thing...)."*

Amazing how insulted some people get when you won't oblige them by eating (or drinking). Don't fret. Better they walk away unhappy than you. And chances are, people who are healthy won't take offense at your demurral.

Frozen

BARRIER: *Stop Journaling*
           Stop Exercising

SOLUTION: *Check That Urge To Check Out, Give Up, Give In*

Often, people stop journaling when they reach their goal weight. They stop noting portion size, quality of their nutrition and before long; they've put the weight back on.

Even – especially – during weight maintenance, you need to continue writing down and therefore monitoring both your food and exercise. As discussed in Chapter TWO, statistically, you're more likely to succeed if you keep a journal. **The principles work as long as you work them; they don't magically work when you stop.**

Another error: people think that as soon as they go on vacation or outside their normal routine, they don't need to journal. In fact, just the opposite is true. In these situations, you need to be more not less conscious (and that means journal). Most likely you'll have less control over your food or your routine. Planning and forethought are even more crucial. **Think of your journal as a soul mate. It goes where you go.** In the best of circumstances, it becomes a part of you.

People often feel that if they're not eating healthily, for example, on holidays or a vacation, why exercise? On those occasions, it's even more important. As long as you are having that extra drink every night, why not take an extra loop around the track, or bike into town instead of drive. **Additional exercise can only add to the pleasure of your vacation, not detract from it.**

Also, better to maintain your exercise routine at a slower rate than abandon it altogether. **It's much easier to keep a habit going than to restart it.** When on vacation (or out of your routine), take advantage of the opportunity to try something different. Aside from the mental excitement, a new sport or activity provides your body with different stimuli and will produce great results. Athletes call this cross-training, and employ it on a regular basis. It enhances performance and speeds recovery (See Chapter TEN).

In short:

- **Keep journaling regardless of where you are in terms of your goals.**

- **Continue your workouts even if your eating is off track. Whatever you do, don't stop.**

> **"Victory belongs to the most persevering."**
> ~Napoleon Bonaparte

Recognizing Your Individual Behaviours

The Change4Good Behaviour GPS© described earlier in the chapter should help you identify your worst triggers and most formidable barriers. Use the chart on the next page to list them in order to identify those behaviours and develop the strategies you need to use to overcome them.

Sample Change4Good Behaviour/Barrier/Strategy Sheet©

Behaviour to Change	My Barriers to Success	My Strategies for Change
Disorganized	Poor time management	Prioritize activities for the day and schedule into daytimer.
Poor sleep habits	Irregular sleep patterns and lack of energy	Watch only one rerun of Gray's Anatomy. Read for 30 minutes. Then go up to bed.
Clean plate syndrome	Eating food because it is there	Ask server for a foil wrapper with dinner. Divide steak in two before eating and wrap other half for tomorrow's dinner.

Your Change4Good Behaviour/Barrier/Strategy Sheet©

Behaviour to Change	My Barriers to Success	My Strategies for Change

You can also download this chart at **www.change4good.ca.**

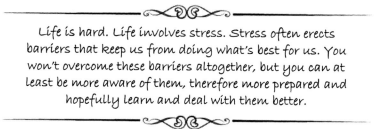

Life is hard. Life involves stress. Stress often erects barriers that keep us from doing what's best for us. You won't overcome these barriers altogether, but you can at least be more aware of them, therefore more prepared and hopefully learn and deal with them better.

Re-read this chapter as often as you like; soon, the principles in it will become a part of your being.

"When you lose, don't lose the lesson."

~Dalai Lama

CHANGE4GOOD – ACTION STEPS

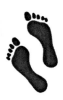

- Start implementing Principle 3 – Identify Barriers; Surmount them.

- Complete your Change4Good Behaviour GPS©.

- Identify 3-5 of your behaviours contributing to your barriers or obstacles and develop strategies to overcome or cope with them.

- Identify and complete your second short-term (weekly) goal. For example: "I will run with friends and *then* go out for a drink" (not no run and three drinks).

- Update Change4Good Journal© daily.

- Update Change4Good Goal Sheet© weekly.

TOOLS

- Change4Good Goal Sheet©

- Change4Good Journal©

- Change4Good Barrier GPS©

- Change4Good Time Journal©

- Change4Good Behaviour/Barrier/Strategy Sheet©

REMEMBER THIS

- Identifying obstacles is half the battle; implementing strategies to overcome them is the other half. When you're done, congratulate yourself. You've run the longest mile.

Change Your Nutrition

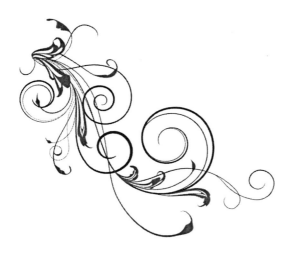

NO NONSENSE NUTRITION: THE BIG THREE, PLUS

This chapter is about the macronutrients; protein, carbohydrates
(good natural ones with fibre) and healthy fats.
Every meal should have them.

Principle 4 Eat Well: *Lean Protein, Natural*
Carbohydrates and Healthy Fats at Each Meal

Taken *ensemble*, the big three (plus fibre) will: slow down the rate
of digestion; keep you fuller longer; give you sustained energy;
stabilize your blood glucose levels and mood, and, in the right
portions, cause you to release less insulin and store less fat – a win-
win proposition. No sane food plan should be without some form of
this guideline.

"Let food be thy medicine."
~Hippocrates

NUTRITION BASICS

You've heard the phrase: you are what you eat. In fact, you are what you digest and absorb, which isn't quite identical to what you eat, but for now, what you eat is a good starting point.

Nutrition determines not only the health and quality of your body – it affects your mind and soul as well. Eating natural, fresh and whole foods in the right proportions and during the right periods throughout the day will help keep you physically healthy and mentally alert and functional.

People think they know about nutrition. And with the flood of articles pouring out over the internet, some do. But many do not. Armchair nutritionists often extract "healthy tips" out of context. Or they adopt rules that don't really apply to their situation. The corporate audiences I've addressed constantly remind me that despite the flurry of information, many remain clueless. In fact, some extremely successful executives don't know the difference between a carbohydrate and a protein. Even athletes can be nutritionally deaf.

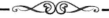

Eating natural, fresh and whole foods in the right proportions and during the right periods throughout the day will help keep you physically healthy and mentally alert and functional.

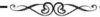

Recently I read the food journal of a client who believed she was doing everything right. I was stunned.

- First, she ate every two hours – too often to give her body a chance to burn calories.
- Second, her carbohydrates were all processed: fat-free puddings, low-fat cinnamon raisin muffins, a sugar-infested "health" cereal and liters of diet soda.
- The first time of day in which she even touched a protein was 5:30p.m. No wonder she was hungry all day. She protested, "But I ate a fibre bar. " "You might as well eat a chocolate bar" was my response. Marketing masquerades as "healthy" what is really a lot of candy-in-disguise.

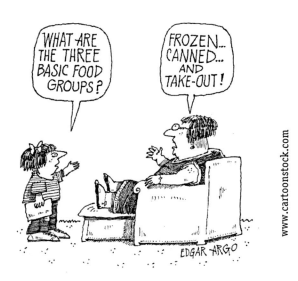

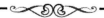

Remember: knowledge is power. Once you know the rudimentary elements – how what you eat affects every living cell – you're much less inclined to abuse yourself by ignoring them.

Nutrition 101

For starters, your body needs nine classes of nutrients for optimal health: two micronutrients (vitamins and minerals), three macronutrients (proteins, carbohydrates and fats), and four other entities (water, enzymes, fibre and antioxidants).

Some of these nutrients are essential (for example water, most vitamins and minerals, certain amino acids and fats), meaning they must be supplied by food as your body cannot produce enough of them to meet the body's needs. The other nutrients are critical for your optimal health and well-being but are not essential because the body can either produce them or survive without them.

Here are nine basic nutrients-that your body needs:

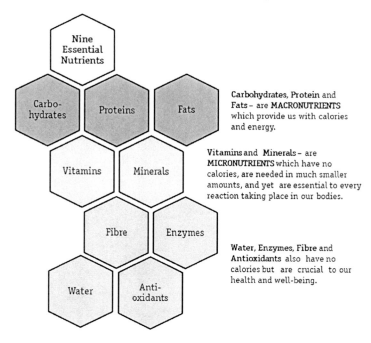

Carbohydrates, Protein and Fats – are MACRONUTRIENTS which provide us with calories and energy.

Vitamins and Minerals – are MICRONUTRIENTS which have no calories, are needed in much smaller amounts, and yet are essential to every reaction taking place in our bodies.

Water, Enzymes, Fibre and Antioxidants also have no calories but are crucial to our health and well-being.

Principle 4 suggests we include all three macronutrients (carbohydrates, protein and fats) in each meal. You don't have to include all three in every snack (although that would be ideal) but try to include at least two. For example, fruit and almonds or cheese and walnuts.

CARBOHYDRATES

Most people adore carbohydrates and no wonder. They're the fun foods that most of us are loath to give up. They're our source of quick energy; also mood-changers, although not always in a healthy way. We'll explore this farther along as we discuss types of carbohydrates.

 But first, the essentials:

- All carbohydrates are broken down into sugar or glucose. (This process occurs regardless of whether you eat a Hostess Twinkie© or a sweet potato).

- Limited amounts are stored as glycogen in the blood, liver and muscles. (Glycogen is the storage form of glucose).

- Excess carbohydrates consumed and not used are stored as body fat. (Same is true of excess fat or protein).

- Carbohydrates are the body's preferred source of fuel to create useable physical and mental energy. (Preferred means more quickly and easily available).

- Carbohydrates are the essential and only fuel for our brain and nervous system.

- Carbohydrates are also a source of fibre which, among other things, keeps us feeling fuller longer.

- Carbohydrates, especially fruits and vegetables, have a high water content, which contributes to our daily intake.

- **The healthiest sources of carbohydrates are fruits, vegetables, legumes and 100% whole grains,** which are packed with essential vitamins, minerals, antioxidants and enzymes.

See page 113 and 114 for a list of carbohydrates recommended on the Change4Good Program. For a complete and regularly updated list, including certain brands, download the Change4Good Grocery List© at **www.change4good.ca.**

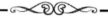

The healthiest sources of carbohydrates are fruits, vegetables, legumes and 100% whole grains, which are packed with essential vitamins, minerals, antioxidants and enzymes.

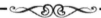

Types of Carbohydrates

The carbohydrates Change4Good wants you to eat are natural carbohydrates in their most natural state.

In other words, **fruits, vegetables** and **100% whole grains** – not processed pears (in syrup), processed vegetables (corn in cream sauce, artificially flavoured mashed potatoes) or processed grains (sugary cereals in spite of whatever *"healthy"* grains are mixed in with the onslaught of sugar and chemicals).

Legumes, which include beans, peas and lentils, are also carbohydrates but have enough protein that vegetarians consider them in the protein category as well.

Many restrictive "diets" mistakenly omit grains. Don't heed them. Grains have nutrients that some fruits and vegetables lack.

To distinguish among carbohydrates is to categorize them as either simple natural; simple processed/refined or complex natural carbohydrates.

The charts below and on the following pages show you how these carbohydrates are different.

Simple Natural Carbohydrates	Contain either one sugar molecule (glucose, fructose, galactose = monosaccharides) or two sugar molecules (sucrose, lactose, maltose = disaccharides).
	Includes: all fruits and non-complex/starchy vegetables, milk, honey, table sugar and malt sugar. Fruits and vegetables are the healthiest sources of simple carbohydrates – they are high in fibre, vitamins, minerals, enzymes, water and antioxidants.
	They are digested relatively quickly, except for fruits and vegetables, which are digested more slowly because of their fibre content.
	Fruits and vegetables are high in fibre which is essential for proper elimination of waste from the body.
	Fruits and vegetables are mostly lower in calories than complex/starchy carbohydrates.

Complex Natural Carbohydrates	Contain three or more sugar molecules (starches = polysaccharides).

Includes: *whole grains (amaranth, brown rice, buckwheat, millet, oatmeal, , wheat germ); breads and cereals made from 100% whole grains; **beans, **lentils, **chickpeas and vegetables like potatoes, yams, sweet potatoes, squash etc.

Take longer to digest than simple carbohydrates and provide a more consistent blood sugar level rise, keeping energy, mood and insulin levels more stable.

Are high in fibre which is essential for proper elimination of waste from the body.

Are more calorie dense than simple carbohydrates like fruit and non-complex/starchy vegetables.

*People sensitive to gluten should stick to the more common gluten-free grains: quinoa, corn, millet, buckwheat and rice.

**Vegetarians should regard legumes as a source of protein. |
| **Simple Refined/Processed Carbohydrates** | Processed and refined carbohydrates are examples of unhealthy, simple carbohydrates that contain empty calories and rob the body of nutrients such as B vitamins, chromium and zinc.

They are easily digested and converted to glucose, move quickly into your blood stream causing blood glucose levels to rise and fall rapidly which influences the release of insulin, a fat storage hormone.

They stress the pancreas and without the proper vitamins and minerals to facilitate metabolism, they are converted to fat, stored in adipose tissue and can increase low-density lipoprotein cholesterol (LDL) levels.

Refined carbohydrates (pastries, refined breads, cookies, pop, etc.) suppress the immune system, are linked to inflammatory conditions, lead to obesity, fatigue, irritability, sugar cravings, mood swings, depression, overeating and anxiety. |

FIBRE

Fibre isn't one of the three macronutrients (carbohydrate, protein and fat but since it's only present in carbohydrates, I discuss it here). In short, fibre is the indigestible cellulose of plants. It's not essential – you could possibly live without it – but not healthily.

It not only helps with regularity, but also lowers your risk of certain diseases. All foods that are high in fibre generally contain two types: soluble and insoluble.

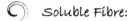 Soluble Fibre:

> This type helps regulate the absorption of both carbohydrates and fats; among its other virtues, it helps lower cholesterol and control blood sugar levels. Soluble fibre does not help with regularity.
>
> **Examples of foods high in soluble fibre include legumes, oats, oat bran, barley, beans, peas, fruit (apples, bananas, citrus fruits), and vegetables (peas, carrots, etc.).**

Insoluble Fibre:

> Also referred to as roughage, it helps move food through your digestive system. It's called 'insoluble' because instead of dissolving (in water), it leaves your body in the form of waste. Insoluble fibre keeps us regular and helps prevent colon cancer.
>
> **Examples of foods high in insoluble fibre include wheat bran, wheat germ, bran cereals, whole grain breads** (100 percent is best; **fibre content should be at least 4-5g a serving to be useful), brown rice, rye and most vegetables.**

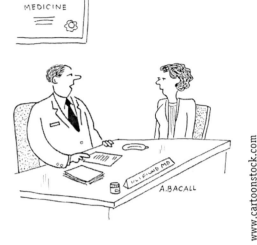

"You need more fiber and less cholesterol in your diet. Throw out the eggs you bought and eat the carton they came in."

How much fibre do you need?

The amount of fibre needed varies depending on age and gender. **A good rule of thumb, however, is: 25 grams for adult women; 38 grams for adult men.** Let's look at an average day's food plan that would provide women with the minimum amount of fibre (men can simply add quantities):

Breakfast • ¼ cup (dry) steel cut oats (4 grams) with 1 scoop protein powder

Snack • 1 medium apple (4 grams) with 10 almonds (1 gram)

Lunch • 1 can tuna with 1 cup raw spinach salad (2 grams) and large sweet potato (6 grams)

Snack • 1/2 cup blueberries (2 grams) and 1/2 cup plain Greek yogurt

Dinner • 3oz grilled salmon with 3/4 cup frozen vegetables (3 grams)

Snack • 1 cup pineapple (2 grams)

TOTAL = 24 grams

If you need to add fibre to your food plan, increase it gradually. Also, be sure to drink plenty of water to help the extra fibre move through the body.

Fruits and vegetables are a great source of fibre. To get more into your diet:

- Try different vegetables and fruits each week.

- Add vegetables such as lettuce, sprouts and tomatoes to sandwiches.

- Add extra vegetables to soups.

- Make vegetable kebabs.

- Buy ready-to-eat vegetables and salads.

- Stock up on frozen vegetables.

- Keep fruits and vegetables where you can see them (eye candy).

- Prepare vegetables ahead of time – wash, cut and store in refrigerator.

- Develop food preparation strategies; they'll help overcome your resistance. A plate of washed cherry tomatoes, snow peas and peeled baby carrots are as easy to eat – and as colourful — as M&Ms©. I keep a giant bowl of cut up peppers, baby carrots, asparagus and cucumbers in my refrigerator at all times. (After all, lettuce does get boring). At meal times, I simply grab a handful to stir-fry or include in a salad and add it to my dinner.

There's never an excuse for not eating vegetables.

⟲ *How much carbohydrate do you need?*

- **Carbohydrates provide 4 calories per gram.**
- **15 grams is considered a serving of carbohydrate** (more on serving sizes in Chapters SIX and SEVEN).
- We should include a combination of the following per day:
    - 2-3 fruit servings (small apple, 1 cup blueberries).
    - At least 3 cups, but ideally 4-6 cups non-starchy vegetables (asparagus, broccoli, cauliflower, kale, mushrooms, onions, string beans, peppers, tomato, etc.). It is because these nutrient dense vegetables are low in carbohydrate content and calories that they can be added freely to any meal or snack.
    - 1 starchy vegetable/legume serving (winter squash, peas, corn, chick peas, pinto beans).
    - 1-2 whole grain servings (1/2 cup oats, millet, barley, brown rice; 1 slice 100% whole grain bread).
- The total amount and type of carbohydrates you eat will depend on:
    - **Body type**
    - **Activity level**
    - **Goals in terms of fat loss**

Depending on these factors, a person who isn't terribly active and wants to lose weight should de-emphasize the calorie-dense carbohydrates (sweet potatoes, rice, green peas, corn and pasta – even whole grains) –and emphasize the less calorie-dense ones (broccoli, string beans, strawberries, apples, even watermelon).

Dr. John Berardi, Ph.D. (nutrition and fitness guru); believes that body type also determines how much and when you should eat carbohydrates. According to this theory each body type has a different carbohydrate tolerance:

○ Ectomorphs:
- Are generally the most carbohydrate-tolerant and can eat a greater percentage of starchy carbohydrates overall and throughout the day.
- They typically have a fast metabolism and find it hard to gain muscle, and they generally lose fat easily.
- They usually have long thin limbs, lean, a small frame and bone structure, small joints and shoulders, stringy muscles and are lean.

○ Mesomorphs:
- Have a more moderate carbohydrate tolerance and should limit their starchy carbohydrate intake to the mornings and/or after workouts.
- The remainder of their meals or snacks should consist of less dense carbohydrates such as non-starchy vegetables and fruits, nuts, seeds and lean protein.
- They typically gain muscle and fat more easily than ectomorphs.
- They usually have a large bone structure, large muscles, are strong with a naturally athletic physique.

○ Endomorphs:
- Are not very carbohydrate-tolerant; they should limit starchy carbohydrates to post-workout meals only.
- The remainder of their meals or snacks should consist of less dense carbohydrates such as non-starchy vegetables and fruits, nuts, seeds and lean protein.
- They typically have a slow metabolism, gain fat easily and struggle to los it; and they can also struggle to gain muscle mass.
- They usually have a short, stocky build, with thick arms and legs, strong muscles especially the upper legs, but overall are soft and round.[7]

Keep in mind that these body types are not set in stone; most of us are a combination of two body types: either ectomorph/mesomorph or mesomorph/endomorph, etc.

 Which are you?

Check the previous list of characteristics, or answer the following questions: How easy is it for you to put on muscle? How do you look at your ideal weight?

Note: Just because a person is thin, doesn't mean they're an ectomorph. My weight qualifies me as being thin but I'm really an endomorph. It's easy for me to put on weight and difficult for me to lose it. I also have to work hard to put on muscle. Essentially I'm a thin person with the body type of someone much heavier; I also have the potential to get heavy quite easily.

- Regardless of your body type, our bodies definitely handle starchy carbohydrates best during and immediately after exercise.
- Also remember that regardless of when and how much carbohydrate you eat, you always need to eat regular meals and snacks throughout the day (Principle 5).

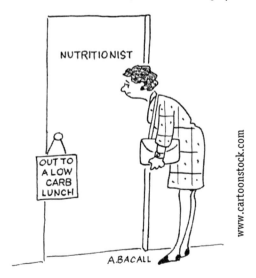

NO NONSENSE NUTRITION: THE BIG THREE, PLUS FIBRE

GLYCEMIC INDEX and GLYCEMIC LOAD

Glycemic Index and Glycemic Load are standards that indicate the body's response to insulin after ingesting a food that contains carbohydrates.

One of the functions of insulin is to regulate blood sugar levels. Too high or too low can have dire consequences (diabetes or hypoglycemia, for example).

The other function of insulin is as a hormone that facilitates the transport of fat (triglycerides) into the fat cells. In this way, it enables our bodies to store fat and therefore increase weight and percentage of body fat – neither of which we want.

Below is a diagram of our body's response to high-glycemic foods, and the subsequent cycle that takes place.

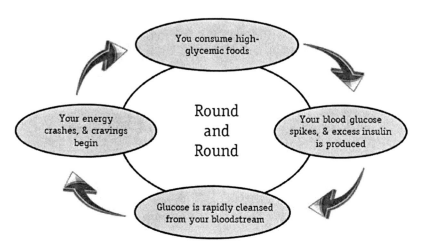

What is the Glycemic Index?

The Glycemic Index ranks carbohydrate foods on how quickly they affect your blood glucose levels. The index measures how much your blood glucose increases after eating 50 grams of a particular carbohydrate.

The ranges for GI are as follows:

Low:	0 – 55
Medium:	56 – 69
High:	70+

 What is the Glycemic Load?

The Glycemic Load of a carbohydrate food is more useful; it takes into account how many grams of carbohydrate are in a typical serving size as well as the GI of that particular carbohydrate. For example, two carbohydrates may have the same GI levels, but the average serving size of one may contain many more grams of carbohydrate than the average serving size of the other, and therefore will affect blood glucose levels differently.

The ranges for GL are as follows:

Low:	0 – 10
Medium:	11 – 19
High:	20+

Sample Comparison of Glycemic Index and Glycemic Load [8]

Food	GI	GL
1 medium raw apple (15 g.)	38	6
6 spears of asparagus (4 g.)	8	1
1 cup brown rice cooked (33 g.)	55	18
1 medium orange (11 g.)	42	5
1 cup spaghetti, whole wheat boiled (37 g.)	37	14
1 cup raw carrots (6 g.)	47	3
1 medium banana (26 g.)	51	14
1 oz. cashew nuts (9 g.)	22	2
2 oz. dried dates (40 g.)	103	42
½ cup boiled green beans (5 g.)	28	1
1 cup dried boiled kidney beans (25 g.)	28	7
1 cup oatmeal (28 g.)	58	16
8 oz. skim milk (13 g.)	32	4
1 cup steamed spinach (7 g.)	6	2
1 cup boiled pearled barley (42 g.)	25	11
1 medium baked russet potato (30 g.)	76	23
½ cup boiled green peas (6 g.)	48	3
1 cup steamed broccoli (4 g.)	6	2
1 ear corn on the cob (29 g.)	53	15
1 cup raw cabbage (7 g.)	6	1
1 cup raw tomato (5 g.)	6	1

**Note: The number of grams indicated in the brackets, represent the carbohydrate amount per serving.

Things to consider:

- The consumption of high glycemic foods raises insulin and reduces glucagons, a situation in which fats can't burn as the body cannot access fat as a fuel source when it contains high levels of insulin.

- Low to moderately glycemic foods break down more slowly, releasing glucose gradually into our bloodstreams and therefore causing a lower and more stable release of insulin.

- The glycemic value of a carbohydrate food only applies if that food is eaten in isolation with no other macro-nutrients. For example, the GI or GL level of rice is useful to know if you're only eating a meal of plain rice. But if you add flax seed oil to the rice, and accompany it with a steak and a salad, the digestion of the carbohydrate in the rice is slowed down by the protein and fat in the meal and its glycemic value is no longer as relevant; it no longer affects blood sugar as it would if it were eaten alone.

- GI and GL are important factors to consider for anyone who wants to maintain a healthy weight and body composition. For diabetics, however, it is especially crucial to monitor how their blood sugar levels are affected by all the foods eaten at a meal.

- Just to complicate matters, not all low glycemic foods are nutritious, and many high glycemic foods are, in fact, nutrient-dense.

  For example, pound cake, low-fat ice cream and peanut M&Ms have a low GI and aren't very nutrient dense whereas millet, watermelon and broad beans have high GIs and are very nutrient dense.

  A food with a low GI and GL is ice cream (not nutrient dense); whereas couscous and dates have high GIs and GLs and are very nutrient dense.

- Glycemic values are also affected by the ripeness of a fruit or vegetable and whether it is cooked or raw. A very ripe banana, for example, will have a higher glycemic value than a green banana; cooked carrots will have a higher glycemic value than raw carrots.

In conclusion, despite criticism and limitations in these indices, there is definitely a correlation between high glycemic diets and chronic diseases such as obesity, type 2 diabetes, cardiovascular disease and certain cancers.

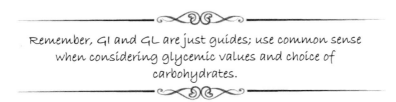

Remember, GI and GL are just guides; use common sense when considering glycemic values and choice of carbohydrates.

SUGAR ALCOHOLS

Another kind of carbohydrate is sugar alcohol, also known as a "polyol." Part of the chemical structure of polyols resembles sugar, and part resembles alcohol – hence the name.

Some sugar alcohols occur naturally in plants and are extracted from them. Most sugar alcohols, however, are manufactured from sugars and starches. Examples include Mannitol, Sorbitol and Xylitol.

Dieters are especially familiar with these sugar alcohols because:

- They're sweet.

- They have approximately 1.5-3 calories per gram, slightly less than regular carbohydrates.

- They are used primarily in low-carbohydrate products because they have less of an impact on blood sugar levels than more natural sugars and because our body cannot completely absorb them.

For this reason, mannitol and sorbitol are often recommended for diabetics. Because sugar alcohols also resist breakdown by bacteria in the mouth, they're less likely to cause tooth decay. In fact, Xylitol may actually prevent tooth decay.

To date, these sweeteners, the newest on the market, have good safety records and few reports of adverse side effects. However, because they are not completely digested in the body, fermenting in the intestines can cause gas, bloating and diarrhea.

Any foods that contain sugar alcohols such as sorbitol or mannitol must include a warning on their labels that states: "Excess consumption may have a laxative effect." The Mayo Clinic suggests that this amount can vary from between 10-50 grams.[9]

Some sources also report increased cravings, caloric intake, insulin levels and weight gain associated with higher amounts of these sweeteners in the diet.

ASPARTAME AND SUCRALOSE

The safety of artificial sweeteners continues to be a controversial topic in both the medical and nutrition community. The more well-known artificial sweeteners include aspartame (NutraSweet®, Equal®) and sucralose (Splenda®).

Although the debate regarding the safety of aspartame in particular appears to be the most contested, with most health complaints relating to the brain and nervous system (headaches, dizziness, anxiety attacks, depression, etc.), sucralose is not much better.

Sucralose should not be confused with sucrose which is table sugar. Although it is made from sugar, it is nothing like sugar and is certainly not natural even though marketing implies that is. The most dangerous ingredient in sucralose is chlorine. Sucralose seems to be associated with fewer adverse health reactions than aspartame, but it has also been on the market for a shorter time with fewer total studies and lack of long term studies on its safety.

In terms of weight management, numerous research studies including amongst others; the Nurse's Health Study[10] and a study completed by The American Cancer Society[11] show that artificial sweeteners may induce sugar cravings, do not promote weight loss and may even cause weight gain.

In the Change4Good program; which avoids processed foods, the general rule regarding artificial sweeteners of any type is: avoid.

STEVIA – A NATURAL SWEETENER

- Stevia is an herb from a plant indigenous to tropical and sub-tropical regions of North and South America.

- It is a natural sweetener that sweetens with almost zero calories.

- Stevia does not encourage cavities.

- It is non-glycemic and is safe for diabetics and may even strengthen the pancreas.

- It is a natural alternative to both artificial sweeteners and sugar.

- The sweetness of stevia is due to phytochemicals called glycosides – the most abundant of these is Stevioside which is over two-hundred times sweeter than sucrose.

- It's available in powder or liquid form; the powder may be used in nearly any kind of recipe, with modifications; the liquid extract is used mainly in beverages.

- One teaspoon of powdered stevia has roughly the same sweetening power as 1 cup of granulated cane sugar and one drop of stevia is roughly equivalent to one teaspoon of sugar.

- Unlike aspartame and sucralose, no known adverse effects have been associated with its use.

If there is a downside of using stevia, it is merely that you continue to anchor yourself to the realm of sweets. Food tastes delicious even when it isn't sweet.

Sometimes, avoiding sweeteners altogether allows you to taste the true flavor of the food. Try your yogurt and berries without stevia once in a while. You may find you don't need it.

Below is a list of healthy carbohydrates. For a complete and regularly updated list, including certain brands, download the Chang4Good Grocery List© at **www.change4good.ca.**

Change4GoodCarbohydrate List©

	Gluten Free Grains	Regular Grains
Grains	buckwheat, corn, kasha, millet, quinoa, rice (basmati, brow, wild)	bran, couscous, hemp, kamut, rye, spelt, steel cut oats, wheat germ
Cereal	cereal – multi/wholegrain	

Change4GoodCarbohydrate List©

Pasta	noodles – soba, tofu	pasta – rice, spinach, whole wheat
Breads	Ezekiel, farmers rye, kamut, spelt, wholegrain, pumpernickel	wholegrain crackers
Dairy	cow's milk (skim, 1%, 2%)	natural, unsweetened almond milk, hemp milk, rice milk
Fruits	fruit - dried (limit), fresh, frozen	
Vegetables	vegetables – fresh, frozen sea vegetables – kelp, nori and dulse	vegetable burgers V-8 Juice®
Legumes	dried, canned (in moderation)	black beans, chickpea, kidney beans, lentils, soy beans, split peas, etc.
Snacks	dark chocolate, fruit cups, hummus and flatbread, popcorn, snack bars, whole grain cookies & muffins, whole grain waffles	
Sweeteners & Spreads	agave nectar, apple sauce, maple syrup, natural jam, raw cane sugar, stevia, unpasteurized honey	

PROTEIN

 A Primer:

- Proteins are the building blocks of the body; they are the second largest percentage of material in the body (water is the first) and are found in every cell in the body.
- Protein is made up of a combination of twenty different amino acids — amino acids are the building blocks of proteins.
- Our bodies can produce eleven of the twenty amino acids, but the other nine, which are called essential amino acids, can only be obtained from specific foods or combinations of foods.
- Food contains two different types of proteins, complete and incomplete proteins.
- **Essential amino acids are found in all complete protein foods**, which include all animal products, as well as soy, quinoa, hemp (and spirulina).
- **We need these complete proteins with all the essential amino acids to support growth and the normal maintenance of all body tissues.**
- **Non-essential amino acids are found in various amounts and combinations in both complete and incomplete protein foods.**
- **Incomplete protein foods** include grain products, nuts, seeds and legumes – they contain some but not all the essential amino acids.
- **By properly combining plant proteins and whole grains (e.g. lentils and rice, i.e. grains and beans) you'll provide your body with the essential amino acids it needs.**

- Whole grains matched with legumes complement each other; each providing the amino acids the other lacks. However, you don't need to do your food combining at one meal; combining these partially complete proteins during the course of a day is sufficient.

Why do you need protein?

- Protein is required for the growth, maintenance and repair of all body tissues.

- It is vital during pregnancy, lactation and early childhood.

- Protein is required for the formation of enzymes and many hormones that regulate our metabolism such as thyroid hormones and insulin.

- Our immune system requires protein, especially for the formation of antibodies that help fight infection.

- Haemoglobin, our oxygen carrying red-blood-cell molecule is a protein.

- Protein controls fluid and salt balance, and acid-alkaline balance.

- Protein also slows down the digestion of a meal and so helps to keep us feeling fuller longer and therefore decreases appetite.

- Protein also helps us burn more calories as the body uses more calories to digest and absorb protein than it does carbohydrates and fats (see Chapter TEN).

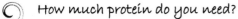

How much protein do you need?

- **Protein, like carbohydrates, also provides 4 calories per gram.**

- **30 grams is equal to one serving** (more on serving sizes in Chapters SIX and SEVEN).

- You should have at least 3 servings of protein per day but ideally, with every meal/snack.

- Dr. John Berardi, Ph.D., a renowned fitness and nutrition expert suggests that all exercising adults should consume approximately 1 gram of protein per pound of body weight, unless they have a body fat percentage greater than 20%; and then they should rather aim for one gram of protein per pound of lean body mass.[12]

- An easier calculation is for **normally active and exercising women to have 20 grams – 30 grams of protein per meal and men, 40 grams – 60 grams per meal.**

- Athletes have different requirements, which need to be calculated on an individual basis based on their body type, sport and goals.

- The American Dietetic Association, Dieticians of Canada and the American College of Sports Medicine all agree that athletes need to consume between 0.5 grams and 0.8 grams of protein per pound of body weight per day.[13]

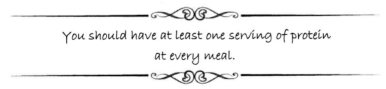

You should have at least one serving of protein at every meal.

Protein for increasing muscle mass:

- Protein is also ideal after a strength-training workout. It helps with muscle repair and thereby helps increase muscle mass. Without extra protein after weight training, muscle growth and repair are compromised.

- However, the belief that eating large amounts of protein will build muscle is not true. Strength training stimulates muscle growth. People engaged in strenuous activity may require more protein but they require more nutrient-dense calories too, including fats and carbohydrates.

- The need for macronutrients and the ratio in which they're required varies, again, depending on body type, activity and goals.

- Amino acids in the blood will stimulate protein synthesis if necessary. **If protein synthesis is not required, the extra protein a person consumes will either be converted into fat** or stored in the body like an excess of any other kind of macronutrient, or it will be converted into toxic ammonia. The body converts this ammonia into urea, which the kidneys then excrete.

- Excess protein can potentially strain the kidneys, which is one reason high protein diets are not recommended.

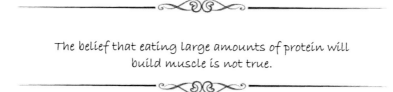

The belief that eating large amounts of protein will build muscle is not true.

Additional tips about healthy sources of protein:

- It is best to consume protein low in saturated fat. Plant foods low in saturated fat that are also complete proteins, as mentioned earlier, are soy, quinoa and hemp.
- Choose plain fat-free Greek yogurt over regular yogurt. Regular yogurt has about 8 grams of protein per serving but even plain, also has a relatively high amount of sugar. Plain fat-free Greek yogurt has 15–20 grams of protein per serving and very little sugar.
- Eat organic products wherever possible (see Chapter NINE).
- Grass-fed animals also produce superior protein.
- Incomplete vegetable sources of protein such as legumes (which included beans, peas and lentils) should be included in the diet.
- High quality protein powders are also a convenient source of protein. Look for protein powders that have the following technical terms:
  - Isolate: gram for gram isolates contain more protein and are purer than concentrates.
  - Cold- filtered: to maximize nutrient integrity.
  - Cross flow micro-filtered: to keep it more pure for the best quality powder.
  - Then choose between whey, casein or hemp (all complete proteins).
  - All should have no artificial sweeteners.

Whey protein best assists with muscle growth and repair and as is ideal after a strength training workout. Casein protein is better at suppressing hunger as it is absorbed more slowly so is more suitable, for example at night, as a snack. The scoreboard: each has advantages and should be used based on individual goals and timing of intake.

About Seafood

Fish, of course, is an especially valuable source of protein because it tends to be leaner than beef or chicken, and in certain cases, also contains healthy fats. However, these days, buying seafood is risky. Because of years of pollution, most seafood is contaminated with either methyl mercury or polychlorinated biphenyls (pcbs) or both, and these are toxic substances.

Which fish are safe, changes with industry conditions and government regulations. Best to keep tabs by checking with the following websites, which provide updated information as to which fish are healthier to eat:

In the USA: www.thefishlist.org
www.seafoodwatch.org

In Canada: www.seachoice.org

For information specifically on the mercury content in fish:
www.nrdc.org/health/effects/mercury/protect.asp

For information specifically on the mercury content in tuna:
www.nrdc.org/health/effects/mercury/tuna.asp

On the next page is a list of healthy proteins to include in your plan. For a complete and regularly updated list, including certain brands, download the Change4Good Grocery List© at **www.change4good.ca.**

Change4GoodProtein List©

Meat	lean red meat – eye round, top round, round tip, top sirloin, bottom round, top loin, tenderloin	beef jerky
Fish	For low risk, moderate risk and high risk fish refer to the websites on the previous page.	
Poultry	white, skinless chicken or turkey	
Eggs	Omega-3, egg whites	
Cheese	light cottage, feta, goat, mozzarella, ricotta single-portioned cheese	
Yogurt	Greek yogurt – natural, fat free Kefir – natural, fat free	
Protein Powder	* protein only * meal replacement	*should be isolate, cold-filtered, cross flow micro-filtered, with no artificial sweeteners
Vegan	edamame, tempeh	meal replacement powders

FATS

At least a minimum intake of fat is important for healthy eating. **There are three main types of lipids or fats:**

- Triglycerides which include Saturated Fatty Acids
- Monounsaturated Fatty Acids
- Polyunsaturated Fatty Acids

Most foods contain a combination of all three. **There are two other two other categories of fats to discuss:**

- **Phospholipids** of which lecithin is the most common example.
- **Sterols** which include phytosterols (plant sterols and plant stanols), cholesterol and some steroid hormones.

You're probably saying, "Too many complex terms." Don't worry. I wouldn't include them if they didn't all provide the solid grounding in nutrition (which every health and fitness minded person needs). Especially if you or anyone you love has heart disease, it's important to have some familiarity with fat esoterica (things understood only by a select few).

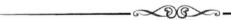

Fat is essential, but it is important to distinguish between those fats that are health-promoting and those that are not.

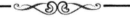

Healthy dietary fat offers protection against heart disease, free radical damage and cancer. According too many nutrition experts, they may even increase metabolic rates and fat burning. **Unhealthy fats, however, are associated with, among other ailments: obesity, cardiovascular disease, diabetes and certain cancers.**

TRIGLYCERIDES: FATS TO LIMIT AND AVOID

Saturated Fats

Saturated fats, along with hydrogenated and trans fats, are the bad fats, the ones you want to avoid. (All three are associated with heart disease, cancer, diabetes and obesity.)

Saturated fats that occur naturally are found most commonly in animal products and certain vegetable oils. They're generally stable and go rancid less easily than mono and polyunsaturated fats.

They are also found in many processed foods, so it's important to always read food labels carefully. (More on that in Chapter SIX).

Examples of saturated fats are: all animal fats (including butter), coconut and palm oils.

Hydrogenated and Trans Fats

Hydrogenated and partially hydrogenated oils or trans fats should be avoided as much as possible. These are unsaturated fats that have been chemically altered for the purpose of making them more stable, improving the texture of baked goods and giving products a longer shelf-life.

In the body, they function like saturated fat but are even more damaging. Trans fats and hydrogenated fats can interfere with the cell's ability to metabolize healthy fats. **They damage cell membranes in a way that keeps out needed nutrients and allows harmful ones to enter, thus setting up the body for chronic, degenerative diseases.** Is it any wonder we should avoid them?

Trans and hydrogenated fats are typically found in margarine, luncheon meats, fried foods, ice cream, cottonseed oil, soybean oil, corn oil, shortening, pastries, cookies and almost all processed foods. Check labels of individual products and avoid any that list trans fats or hydrogenated or partially hydrogenated oils.

HEALTHY FATS: THE UNSATURATED FATS

There are two types of unsaturated fats, monounsaturated and polyunsaturated. They are mostly liquid at room temperature but are also both unstable and sensitive to interaction with oxygen, light and heat. They are best stored in dark containers and refrigerated.

 Monounsaturated Fats (Omega-9)

Our bodies produce monounsaturated fats, which is why although a healthy fat, it is not one of the essential fats. When eaten in moderation and used to replace saturated and trans fats, monounsaturated fats can help lower total cholesterol and LDLs, and raise HDLs – our so-called good cholesterol.

HDL or high density lipoprotein is found in the bloodstream. It returns excess cholesterol from the cells to the liver. LDL or low density lipoprotein transports fats and cholesterol to the cells via the bloodstream. An excess of Omega-9, however, can interfere with essential fatty acid function.

Food sources:

• Examples of foods high in monounsaturated fats include vegetable oils such as olive oil, peanut oil, sunflower oil and sesame oil.
• Other sources of monounsaturated fats are avocados, natural nut butters and many other nuts and seeds.

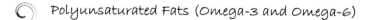 Polyunsaturated Fats (Omega-3 and Omega-6)

Polyunsaturated fats are considered essential fats. Omega-3 (alpha-linolenic acid) and Omega-6 (linoleic acid) are critical to our health in many ways:

- They help to lower blood pressure and cholesterol levels.
- They improve immune system function, fat metabolism, hormone regulation, brain function, normal growth and development.
- They keep our skin healthy, control pain and inflammation, improve mood and even protect us from memory loss in old age. Pretty amazing stuff, right?

However, polyunsaturated fats, alas, cannot be manufactured by the body and must therefore be supplied through diet. They should be consumed in a 2:1 ratio of Omega-6: Omega-3 for optimal health. How you do achieve the proper ratio you may wonder? There isn't any simple answer. However, since most of us get enough Omega-6 through our diet, the key is to concentrate on obtaining sufficient Omega-3.

- **Sources of Omega-6 fats include safflower, sunflower, hemp, walnut, pumpkin, sesame and flax seeds and oils, and borage and evening primrose oils.**

- **Sources of Omega-3 fats include flax, chia, salba, hemp, sacha inchi, pumpkin and walnut seeds and/or oils; cold-water fish such as sardines, salmon, mackerel, trout and fish oil supplements.**

A note on nuts and seeds: in order to benefit from the healthy fats in these foods, make sure they are not roasted, as the heat from roasting destroys the healthy fats in them.

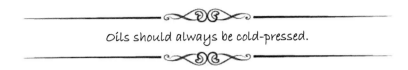

Oils should always be cold-pressed.

EPA and DHA are two Omega-3 oils critical to our health.
(Their full names, in case you are dying to know, are:
eicosapentaenoic acid and docosahexaenoic acid.) Note
that we cannot get either EPA or DHA directly from plant
sources. Our bodies can convert the Omega-3 in plants to
EPA and DHA, but not very effectively. Non-fish eaters
or vegetarians can use flaxseed oil, a plant-based source
of Omega-3 fat, to get their EPA and DHA indirectly, but
whether enough is converted and how efficient the
conversion process is, is a subject of debate.

PHOSPHOLIPIDS

 Lecithin

Phospholipids are chemically similar to triglycerides. They
form part of all cell membranes and help control what
can enter a cell and what can leave it.

Lecithin is a phospholipid that contains both Omega-3
and Omega-6 fats. It is a major structural component of
cell membranes. It contains a substance called choline,
which is needed to make the neurotransmitter
acetylcholine required for proper brain and nerve
function. It also plays a role in certain liver
detoxification functions. In addition, it is an important
part of bile and acts as an emulsifier of fats during
digestion, it keeps cholesterol soluble and isolated from
arterial linings, and it protects it from oxidation. Finally
it also helps prevent and dissolve gall and kidney stones.

Taking lecithin in supplement form (since it is normally found in foods with a high fat content) can benefit people with high cholesterol or heart disease. Some studies also suggest a possible role in improving memory and the slowing of Alzheimer's disease, but the research is inconclusive.

Food sources of lecithin include: egg yolks, wheat germ, peanut butter and soybeans.

STEROLS

Sterols are natural steroids from plants and animals. Plant sterols and stanols belong to a class of naturally occurring plant compounds called phytosterols. Cholesterol is an example of an animal sterol.

 Phytosterols

Both plant sterols and stanols are necessary structural components in plants. They protect the integrity of the cell membrane just as cholesterol does for the cells of the human body.

Sterols and stanols occur naturally in small amounts in many grains, vegetables, fruits, legumes, nuts and seeds.

Plant sterols and stanols have shown to lower total cholesterol and LDL cholesterol (bad cholesterol) without having any effect on HDL (good cholesterol) – more reason to eat healthy, natural foods.

Cholesterol

Cholesterol is perceived as a bad word, primarily due to its implication in the cause of heart disease. However, it is the oxidized cholesterol and LDL in our blood that is the problem. The level of these substances is more a result of a person's genetics than simply the amount of cholesterol in our food and total intake of poor dietary fats (like trans and hydrogenated fats).

Cholesterol, in fact is primarily produced in our bodies from the breakdown of sugars, fats and even protein – especially when our intake of these foods supplies us with excess calories and especially excess sugars and non-essential fatty acids.

In addition, our bodies also make more cholesterol when we are:
   a) Under stress.
   b) Dehydrated.
   c) Suffer from dietary deficiencies of the vitamins and minerals required to metabolize cholesterol.

In short, the cholesterol in the food we eat is just a small part of the way in which cholesterol is associated with heart disease. Cholesterol is found primarily in animal products, most notably in egg yolk.

On the plus side, cholesterol is an important nutrient in our make-up. Manufactured primarily in our liver, it is a component of all our cell membranes. The liver, brain, nervous system and blood have the highest amounts. Our body uses cholesterol to make Vitamin D, estrogen, testosterone, steroid hormones and bile, which are all essential to health.

Steroid Hormones

Our body makes steroid hormones from cholesterol. Examples include: the male and female sex hormones, testosterone and estrogen and progesterone respectively.

The steroids that are often in the news are anabolic steroids, drugs made to mimic the effect of male sex hormones. Health risks associated with excessive or long-term use of these steroids include harmful changes in cholesterol levels, acne, mood swings and both heart and liver damage.

Our body also makes adrenal corticosteroid hormones from cholesterol. An example is aldosterone which regulates water balance via our kidneys.

Why do we need healthy fats?

Although we've mentioned some of the benefits of the healthy fats, here's an overview of why fat is essential to our diet:

- They are a source of fuel for our bodies.
- They are needed to transport the fat-soluble vitamins, vitamins A, D, E and K.
- They are a part of cell membranes.
- They provide organ protection and thermal insulation.
- Omega-3s help control inflammatory responses.
- They are needed for circulation and healthy skin.

- They are involved with weight management, hormone and PMS regulation.
- They make food taste good and create a feeling of satiety (fullness).
- They take relatively long to digest, and therefore help us stay full for a longer period.
- Omega-3s in particular are critical for brain and nervous system function and a healthy immune system; they also help metabolize cholesterol and all fats (or triglycerides).

A Burning Issue: Do Fats Help Us Burn Fat?

Omega-3 fatty acids definitely improve metabolic health but do they actually help us lose body fat and therefore body weight? Numerous studies have been completed over the past decade suggesting that the highly unsaturated Omega-3 fats found in cold water fish called EPA (eicosapentaenoic acid) and DHA (decosahexaenoic acid) may help you lose more fat. However these findings are not conclusive.

In addition, the fat loss benefit doesn't seem all that substantial. Some researchers believe that the improvement in fat loss is merely the result of correcting Omega-3 deficiencies or the balance of Omega-3 and Omega-6, implying that the improvement in fat loss may be short lived.

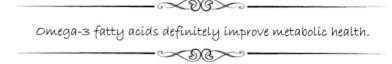

Omega-3 fatty acids definitely improve metabolic health.

Regardless, enough other benefits of eating fatty fish or taking a fish oil supplement have been proven which should encourage you to take in those Omega-3s.

For weight loss, approximately 1–3 teaspoons a day is generally recommended. For strictly nutritional purposes, 1 teaspoon a day is fine for most.

For a list of recommended Omega -3 supplements, you can download the Change4Good Supplements for Health List© at **www.change4good.ca.**

 How much total fat do we need?

- Fat, a more concentrated source of energy than carbohydrates or protein, contains **9 calories per gram.** As a result, we need less of it in our diet.

- Generally we should not get more than **20-35%** of our calories from fat[14], and most of those should come from monounsaturated and polyunsaturated fats.

- **Approximately 5 grams or 1 teaspoon of fat is one serving.** (More on serving sizes in Chapter SIX and SEVEN.)

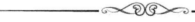

*Generally we should not get more than 20 - 35%
of our calories from fat.*

COOKING WITH FATS

Although **frying is never recommended as a means of cooking**, some oils and fats are definitely safer for frying or cooking at high temperatures (up to 375°F) than others. Saturated fats are more stable and less sensitive to light, heat and air and are therefore best used for high temperature cooking. Butter and ghee are best; other good choices are coconut and palm oil, and other tropical fats.

Fats that are suitable for cooking at medium (up to 325 ° F) to low (up to 212°F) temperatures include, in order of preference, high oleic (monounsaturated) sunflower and safflower oil, peanut oil, sesame oil and olive oil.

A good cooking strategy is to first put water in your frying pan and heat it. Then add oil. This method keeps temperatures down and is therefore, less likely to destroy the oils.

Essential fats such as flax and hemp are extremely sensitive to oxygen, heat and light and should never be heated. High temperatures destroy their beneficial properties and turn them rancid.

Rancidity (the chemical decomposition of fats and oils) promotes the formation of free- radicals, which you do not want. For this reason, **EFAs (essential fatty acids) which are sensitive to heat and light should always be refrigerated in dark coloured containers.** Fats can be kept fresh longest by keeping them: at very cool temperatures, in the dark and unexposed to air or oxygen.

Essential fats are best used in protein shakes, salad dressings, on grilled vegetables and cooked oatmeal.

Below is a list of healthy fats to include in your plan. For a complete and regularly updated list, download the Change4Good Grocery List© at **www.change4good.ca.**

Change4GoodFats List©

Nuts & Seeds	nuts: raw/unsalted almonds, pecans, walnuts, pine nuts etc. butters: almond, cashew, peanut etc.	seeds: raw/unsalted chia, flax, hemp, pumpkin, sacha inchi, salba, sesame, sunflower etc.
Oils	coconut, flax seed, hemp seed, olive – extra virgin, cold-pressed, peanut, pumpkin seed, sesame seed	
Other	avocado butter (unsalted), ghee	cold water fish (sardines, salmon, mackerel, trout)

Now that you have a pretty good understanding of the macronutrients, you'll probably better understand the importance of including all three macronutrients in at least each of the three meals you eat every day (Principle 4). All of them have elements essential for overall health and, when combined at the right time and in the right portions, provide the greatest benefit in terms of health, weight management and sustained energy.

On the following pages are another two days from my personal food journal. These together with my food journals in Chapter TWO should give you plenty of ideas of various food combinations and options for meals and to enable you to see how to practically implement Change4Good Principle 4 - Eat Well: Lean Protein, Natural Carbohydrates and Healthy Fats at Each Meal. (More on timing in Chapter FIVE and on portion control in Chapter SEVEN). In the meantime, eat regularly throughout the day, starting with breakfast followed by a balanced, nutritious meal or snack approximately every three hours. You won't feel hungry and your body will thank you.

Change4Good Journal© - Sample #3

Date: *July 11 2011*	LP: Lean Protein, NC: Natural Carbs, HF: Healthy Fats, O: Other

Weather ☀ ☁ 🌧	Energy Level ⬆ ➡ ⬇	Mood 😊 😐 ☹

Time	Meal/Snack 1: What I Ate	Portion
10:00 a.m.	French toast	
	LP: *Egg whites*	*¾ cup*
	NC: *Ezekiel bread*	*2 slices*
	HF: *Almond butter*	*2 tsp*
	O: *Tea with 2% milk*	.

Weather ☀ ☁ 🌧	Energy Level ⬆ ➡ ⬇	Mood 😊 😐 ☹

Time	Meal/Snack 2: What I Ate	Portion
1:30 pm	Grilled tilapia with brown rice and salad	
	LP: *Grilled tilapia*	*3 oz*
	NC: *Brown rice; green salad (spinach)*	*½ cup, 1 cup*
	HF: *Avocado and low fat salad dressing*	*1/8, 1 tbsp*
	O:	

Weather ☀ ☁ 🌧	Energy Level ⬆ ➡ ⬇	Mood 😊 😐 ☹

Time	Meal/Snack 3: What I Ate	Portion
4:00 pm	Babybel cheese and pineapple	
	LP: *Babybel cheese light*	*2*
	NC: *Pineapple*	*¾ cup*
	HF:	
	O:	

Water	🥛🥛🥛 🥛🥛🥛🥛🥛 🥛🥛🥛🥛🥛 🥛🥛
Supplements	*Omega – 3, Juice Plus, Vitamin D3, Maca Powder*

Change4Good Journal© – Sample #3

LP: Lean Protein, NC: Natural Carbs, HF: Healthy Fats, O: Other

Weather ☀ ⛅ 🌧	Energy Level ↑ ↔ ↓	Mood ☺ 😐 ☹
Time	**Meal/Snack 4: What I Ate**	**Portion**
7:30 pm	Thin multi grain pizza	
	LP: Tuna as topping	½ can
	NC: Pizza base; Mushrooms, onion, spinach, pepper	3 slices, ½ cup
	HF: Olive oil	2 tsp
	O:	

Weather ☀ ⛅ 🌧	Energy Level ↑ ↔ ↓	Mood ☺ 😐 ☹
Time	**Meal/Snack 5: What I Ate**	**Portion**
10:30 pm	Ryvita and ricotta cheese	
	LP: Light ricotta cheese	3 tbsp
	NC: Ryvita crackers	3
	HF:	
	O:	

Weather ☀ ⛅ 🌧	Energy Level ↑ ↔ ↓	Mood ☺ 😐 ☹
Time	**Meal/Snack 6: What I Ate**	**Portion**
	LP:	
	NC:	
	HF:	
	O:	

Workout Summary	Cardio – 45 minute elliptical (8:30 am)

Change4Good Journal© – Sample #4

| Date: July 12 2011 | | LP: Lean Protein, NC: Natural Carbs, HF: Healthy Fats, O: Other | | |

Weather ☀ ☁ 🌧	Energy Level ⬆➡⬇	Mood ☺ 😐 ☹

Time	Meal/Snack 1: What I Ate	Portion
10 am	Protein Shake	
	LP: Protein powder	1 scoop
	NC: Almond milk	½ cup
	HF: Flaxseed oil	1 tsp
	O: Ice	

Weather ☀ ☁ 🌧	Energy Level ⬆➡⬇	Mood ☺ 😐 ☹

Time	Meal/Snack 2: What I Ate	Portion
1:00 pm	Grilled salmon with quinoa and salad	
	LP: Grilled salmon	3 oz
	NC: Quinoa; spinach salad	½ cup, 1 cup
	HF: Salad dressing; olive oil and lemon juice	2 tbsp each
	O:	

Weather ☀ ☁ 🌧	Energy Level ⬆➡⬇	Mood ☺ 😐 ☹

Time	Meal/Snack 3: What I Ate	Portion
4:00 pm	Apple with almond butter	
	LP:	
	NC: Apple	1 medium
	HF: Almond butter	1 tbsp
	O: Tea with 2% milk	

Water	🥛🥛🥛🥛🥛🥛🥛🥛🥛🥛🥛🥛
Supplements	Omega – 3, Juice Plus, Vitamin D3, Maca Powder

Change4Good Journal© – Sample #4

LP: Lean Protein, NC: Natural Carbs, HF: Healthy Fats, O: Other

Weather ☀ ⛅ ☁	Energy Level ↑ ⟷ ↓	Mood ☺ 😐 ☹
Time	**Meal/Snack 4: What I Ate**	**Portion**
7:15 pm	Asparagus mushroom omelette and yam	
	LP: Eggs	2
	NC: Yam, asparagus, mushrooms	1 small, ½ cup
	HF:	
	O:	

Weather ☀ ⛅ ☁	Energy Level ↑ ⟷ ↓	Mood ☺ 😐 ☹
Time	**Meal/Snack 5: What I Ate**	**Portion**
10 pm	Greek yogurt, blueberries, flaxseed and honey	
	LP: Greek yogurt	½ cup
	NC: Frozen blueberries; honey	½ cup, 1 tsp
	HF: Ground flaxseed	1 tbsp
	O:	

Weather ☀ ⛅ ☁	Energy Level ↑ ⟷ ↓	Mood ☺ 😐 ☹
Time	**Meal/Snack 6: What I Ate**	**Portion**
	LP:	
	NC:	
	HF:	
	O:	

Workout Summary	700 Rep Circuit (8.30am)

CHANGE4GOOD – ACTION STEPS

- Start implementing Principle 4 – Eat Well: Lean Protein, Natural Carbohydrates and Healthy Fats at Each Meal.
- Introduce at least two new natural carbohydrates (acorn squash, wheat berries), healthy fats (avocado and sacha inchi seeds) and a plant based protein (hemp, quinoa) into your diet.
- Identify and complete your third short term (weekly) goal. For example: "I will eat fish twice a week; I will trade aspartame for stevia (if I need a sweetener); I will trade margarine for butter or olive oil; I will find or devise great recipes for salad dressing using flaxseed oil." (Mine is in Chapter NINE).
- Update Change4Good Journal© daily.
- Change4Good Goal Sheet© weekly.

TOOLS

- Change4Good Goal Sheet©

- Change4Good Journal©

- Change4Good Grocery List©

REMEMBER THIS

- REMEMBER THIS . . . The absolutely best way to reduce cravings is the simplest: eat lean protein, healthy carbohydrates and healthy fats at every meal.

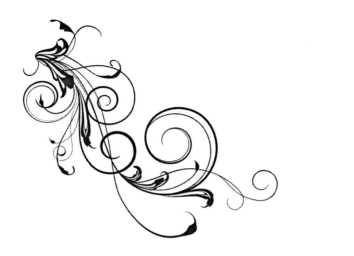

NO NONSENSE NUTRITION – 2:
THE OTHER FIVE, PLUS DIGESTION

This chapter is about the other nutrients that our bodies need (vitamins, minerals, enzymes, water and antioxidants) and the beautiful way in which our bodies digest and absorb them.

Principle 5 Eat Often: 4–6 Nutrient-Dense Meals/Snacks Each Day

The more micronutrients you give your body, the more it will pay you back with good looks, good health and, maybe even happiness. So why waste a meal on nutritionally empty food? In terms of weight management, eating nutrient-dense foods regularly throughout the day will not only nourish your body with what it really needs, but will also help to reduce cravings, manage your hunger and keep your energy and moods sublimely steady.

> **"Things sweet to taste prove in digestion sour."**
> ~William Shakespeare

Let's say you wake up in the morning, and you aren't hungry. Chances are you ate too much the previous night. Spreading your meals and snacks evenly throughout the day, approximately every three hours will ensure at least the following:

- That you eat often enough so as not to become over hungry and overeat; especially later in the day.

- That you don't eat too frequently (as in grazing), preventing your body from burning any stored calories (fat) you have for energy.

- In addition eating too frequently lessens the time our systems and organs have to replace damaged cells and tissue and keep our immune system strong.

However, once you follow Principle 5 - Eat Often: 4–6 Nutrient-Dense Meals/Snack Each Day, you'll find yourself waking in the morning with healthy hunger: a bracing way to start the day.

What you eat during these intervals obviously matters too; **the more nutrient-dense the food, the better. Eating processed junk foods not only harms your health and adds weight; it stimulates your appetite for more junk.** Empty calories leave you feeling hungry and for logical reasons: although you're getting calories, your body isn't getting the nutrients it needs. It's like putting pop or water in the gas tank of your car; the tank may be full but the car won't move.

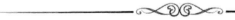

Empty calories leave you feeling hungry and for logical reasons: although you're getting calories, your body isn't getting the nutrients it needs.

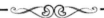

THE OTHER SIX

Now that you know about the big three (protein, carbohydrates, and fat), let's get familiar with the no-less-important other five nutrients: vitamins, minerals, enzymes, antioxidants and of course the life sustaining nutrient, water. (The ninth nutrient, fibre, was discussed in Chapter FOUR; see the carbohydrate discussion). In this chapter, we'll also look at digestion. What good is ingesting all these great nutrients if your body can't absorb them?

There are nine basic nutrients that your body needs:

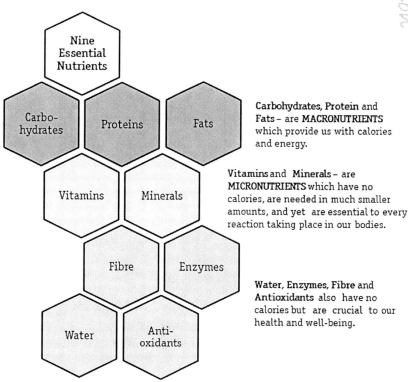

Carbohydrates, Protein and Fats – are **MACRONUTRIENTS** which provide us with calories and energy.

Vitamins and Minerals – are **MICRONUTRIENTS** which have no calories, are needed in much smaller amounts, and yet are essential to every reaction taking place in our bodies.

Water, Enzymes, Fibre and Antioxidants also have no calories but are crucial to our health and well-being.

VITAMINS AND MINERALS

Some 45 known essential nutrients are required in specific
amounts for the body to function properly. As in Chapter
FOUR, the term "essential" means that the body cannot
synthesize the nutrient internally. Therefore all "essential"
nutrients must come from exogenous, or outside, sources.

**In addition to carbohydrates, fats (lipids), complete proteins,
and water, there are at least 14 kinds of vitamins, and at least
20 kinds of minerals required for proper metabolic function** (*at
least* because experts disagree on the exact numbers).

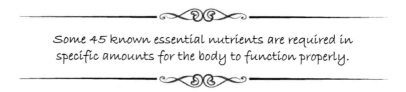

*Some 45 known essential nutrients are required in
specific amounts for the body to function properly.*

VITAMINS:

- **Vitamins along with minerals and enzymes ensure proper
  regulation of just about every physiological process in our
  bodies.** Each vitamin has a specific function or meets one or
  more specific bodily needs.

- Vitamins are not part of our tissue and do not directly
  provide energy but they do **convert the macronutrients in
  our diet into forms that help our body use them.**

- **Vitamins are essential for: growth, the production and
  maintenance of tissues; the maintenance of the immune
  system; protection against cellular damage, and our overall
  vitality and general health.** Typically, each has more than
  one function.

- **Depletions or deficiencies can lead to specific nutritional disorders** as well as general problems, depending on which vitamin is lacking and to what extent.

- **Vitamins are easily destroyed by exposure to light, water, air and heat** (which of course includes cooking and processing). Discussion of raw versus cooked later on in this chapter.

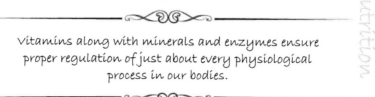

Vitamins along with minerals and enzymes ensure proper regulation of just about every physiological process in our bodies.

- **There are two categories of vitamins: water-soluble vitamins and fat-soluble vitamins:**

  Water-Soluble Vitamins:

  - **B Vitamins**, namely Thiamin, Riboflavin, Niacin, B6, B12, Biotin, Pantothenic Acid, Folate and Choline.

  - **Vitamin C.**

  - Water-soluble vitamins are not stored in our body, and therefore, need to be consumed every day.

  - The B vitamins are typically referred to as a B-complex as they are commonly found together in foods, and have similar co-enzyme functions – meaning they usually need each other to perform optimally.

- The B-Vitamins help provide energy by acting with enzymes to convert carbohydrates to glucose and are also important in fat and protein metabolism.

- They are also crucial to the normal functioning of the nervous system.

- Vitamin C is essential for the formation and maintenance of collagen which is the basic connective tissue found in our skin, ligaments, cartilage and capillary linings.

- Vitamin C is also an antioxidant and stimulates the immune system.

- **B Vitamins are found primarily in vegetables, whole grains, brewer's yeast and molasses; Vitamin C is found in many fruits, especially citrus fruits and vegetables.**

Fat-Soluble Vitamins:

- Vitamin A, D, E, K.

- They are found in the lipid component of both vegetable and animal-source foods.

- They are stored in the body and are not required daily, nutritionally or supplementally.

- Because they are stored, consuming a surplus can cause our supply to reach toxic levels.

- The **primary functions** of the fat-soluble vitamins:

  - Vitamin A helps protect cells as well as resist infection.

  - Vitamin D aids in the absorption of calcium and is also associated with mental wellness, cognitive and immune function.

  - Vitamin K is crucial in blood clotting.

  - Vitamin E functions as a major antioxidant protecting our bodies from the harmful by-products of metabolism and outside pollutants.

MINERALS:

- **Minerals are a basic constituent of all matter.**

- They are part of living tissue but also exist in inorganic forms in the earth.

- **Approximately 4-5 % of our body weight is mineral matter and most of that is our skeleton.**

- Minerals are also found in tissue proteins, enzymes, blood and some vitamins.

- Like vitamins, they also contain no calories and therefore provide no energy themselves, but help:

  - **Produce energy and regulate other body processes.**
  - **Regulate fluid balance and metabolism, form blood, bones and specific chemical messengers.**
  - **Maintain a healthy nervous system.**
  - **Regulate and maintain muscle tone and overall physical development.**

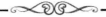

Minerals are a basic constituent of all matter.
Approximately 4-5% of our body weight is mineral
matter and most of that is our skeleton.

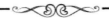

- Our bodies cannot make minerals, which is why we must obtain them through diet.

- Natural minerals come from the earth; if a mineral nutrient isn't found in the soil in which a food is grown, it won't be in that food – another reason to work against industrial or other practices that deplete the nutritional value of the soil.

- The mineral content of food gives each food, when digested and absorbed, the potential for being acidic or alkaline. (The impact of acidity or pH balance is discussed in Chapter NINE).

- A concern with minerals is their rate of absorption by our bodies – even when our digestive system is functioning well, most minerals are only moderately well absorbed.

- Minerals are not destroyed by heat but some are soluble in water and are therefore lost or leached during cooking. Does that mean we should all go raw? If only the answer were that simple.

- Loss of minerals also occurs during food processing.

- Mineral deficiencies can cause major and minor health problems, the most common being osteoporosis in women, and anemia in female competitive athletes and vegans.

The People versus Myths about Nutrition: Raw versus Cooked

There are advantages to eating both cooked and raw foods. Cooking certainly does destroy certain nutrients – Vitamin C, for example, as well as certain enzymes. Myrosinase, an important cancer fighting enzyme, is destroyed when broccoli is steamed.

On the other hand, the digestive tract absorbs certain nutrients more successfully when the foods that contain them are cooked (boiled or steamed). The reason; vegetables are plants; plants are surrounded by a somewhat impervious cell wall that must be broken down to allow maximum absorption of healthy antioxidants, vitamins, and carotenoids. The heat used during cooking helps to break down that wall so that nutrients can be more readily absorbed.

Here are some examples that illustrate this:

- Less of the carotenoids in carrots are absorbed when they're eaten raw, whereas more are absorbed from cooked carrots.
- Cooking also boosts the amount of lycopene in tomatoes: the heat breaks down the plant's thick cell walls and increases the body's uptake of some of the nutrients bound to those walls.
- Spinach, mushrooms, asparagus, cabbage, peppers and many other vegetables also yield more antioxidants, such as carotenoids and ferulic acid, when cooked rather than raw.
- Certain minerals like calcium and magnesium found in leafy greens are also more available if cooked.
- Finally, indole, another important cancer preventative enzyme, is made more readily available through cooking.

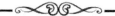

There are advantages to eating both cooked and raw foods.
My verdict; eat both raw and steamed vegetables daily.

How to Preserve All Those Precious Nutrients in Fruits and Vegetables

- **Both fruits and vegetables are highly perishable.** They lose substantial amounts of nutrients as a result of being harvested early, improperly handled and stored for long periods. For this reason, locally grown is often better.

- **Frozen fruits and vegetables, too, can have higher nutrient levels as they are generally harvested at peak ripeness and frozen within a couple of hours.**

- **How you prepare frozen foods affects their nutritional content.** For example, water-soluble vitamins can leach out of the food and dissolve in the cooking water. To preserve as many nutrients as possible, cook vegetables in small amounts of water, and reuse the water for soups and sauces.

- **Avoid thawing frozen vegetables before cooking** as it causes the loss of water that was naturally in the produce which contains some of the water-soluble vitamins.

- **When preparing produce for cooking, cut into larger pieces, thus reducing the surface area exposed to heat and water, and therefore preserving nutrients.**

- **Quick cooking methods like steaming and stir-frying, which involve little contact between the produce and the water, may also conserve nutrients.** The lower the cooking temperature the better; and cook until tender but crisp.

MACRO and MICRO MINERALS:

Macro-minerals, which include calcium, magnesium, phosphorous, sodium, potassium, sulphur and chloride, are needed in larger amounts in the body (more than 100mg/day).

Micro-minerals, which include iron, zinc, copper, cobalt, iodine, selenium, manganese, molybdenum and chromium, are needed in smaller amounts (less than 100mg/day).

Both types are essential for life processes.

 Macro-Minerals:

Calcium:	What our bones and teeth are made of; necessary for blood clotting, muscle contraction, nerve transmission and cell metabolism.
Phosphorous:	Also in our bones and teeth, as well as our DNA and phospholipids (a type of fat; see Chapter FOUR). Phosphorous helps maintain acid/base balance.
Sodium & Potassium:	Maintains fluid balance and transmission of nerve impulses.
Sulphur:	Component of certain amino acids and vitamins.
Chloride:	Maintains fluid balance; helps produce stomach acid, transmits nerve impulses and maintains acid/base balance.
Magnesium:	Needed for many nerve and heart functions.

◯)   Micro-Minerals:

Iron:	Critical component of haemoglobin and myoglobin – both involved in transporting oxygen. There are two forms of iron: heme (found in meat) and non-heme (found in vegetables and grains). Heme iron is the more absorbent form.
Zinc:	Helps activate many enzymes; growth and development; antioxidant activity; immune function and ability to taste.
Copper:	Promotes iron metabolism; is a component of antioxidant enzymes as well as enzymes involved in connective tissue synthesis.
Cobalt:	Part of B12 and essential for red blood-cell formation.
Iodine:	Needed to make thyroid hormone.
Selenium:	Has antioxidant properties and is involved in the normal functioning of the immune system and thyroid gland.
Manganese:	A part of certain enzymes, including some involved in carbohydrate metabolism.
Molybdenum:	A component of certain co-enzymes (which aid enzyme functions).
Chromium:	Enhances the action of insulin.

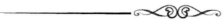

Both macro and micro minerals are essential for life processes.

ENZYMES:

- **Enzymes are proteins produced by our cells that, in turn, facilitate or initiate other chemical reactions.** The chemical reactions inside us depend on them. Without enzymes, these reactions would occur extremely slowly if at all.

- **Enzymes are sensitive to pH, temperature and the presence of certain other vitamins and minerals.** If the pH or temperature is off, enzymes will not function. Raw foods contain enzymes but cooking inactivates or denatures them so that they can no longer assist in the digestion process. (See earlier discussion: Raw vs. Cooked.)

There are three types of enzymes: metabolic, digestive and food enzymes.

- Metabolic Enzymes **are vital to the functioning of every cell.** A short list of some of the chemical reactions they catalyze (cause and speed up) includes:
  - Destroying and removing toxins.
  - Producing energy.
  - Repairing damaged tissues.
  - Strengthening the immune system.

  Enzymes are job-specific: different cells require different enzymes in order to function.

- **Digestive and Food Enzymes have only one main purpose: to digest our food** (i.e., getting it into a state so that it can be absorbed through the walls of the small intestine and released into the blood stream). **There is almost no activity more important to the body than digesting food and turning it into nutrients.**

- **Digestive enzymes** are produced within our bodies. **No food can be digested without digestive enzymes.** Our organs make them. They are secreted by the salivary glands, stomach, pancreas, and the small intestine.

  Examples of some digestive enzymes include protease, which digests protein, lipase which digests fats, amylase which digests carbohydrates, lactase which digests lactose, maltase which digests maltose and sucrose which digests sucrase. Our supply of these enzymes decreases with age.

- **Food Enzymes** exist naturally in raw food; hence we get them from food. **Uncooked, most food contains enough natural food enzymes to greatly assist in digestion.** For example, when we eat a salad, fish and a sweet potato, the food enzymes in the salad help to digest the meal so that we are not relying on as many enzymes from our body to do the work so that the nutrients from the meal can be absorbed by our body. Cooked, the fish and sweet potato don't provide any food enzymes to aid in digestion. Our body, therefore, must internally release the digestive enzymes necessary to handle the task. **The more we depend on internally generated digestive enzymes, the quicker we use up this supply.**

  Raw food certainly provides more enzymes, but remember: in some cases, cooked food provides more nutrients, is easier to digest and absorb and can protect us from food-borne illnesses. Again, the preferred stand: eat both.

ANTIOXIDANTS:

Antioxidants are a group of vitamins, minerals and plant substances. They consist of: phytonutrients, flavonoids and bioflavonoids. **Although not essential, antioxidants have protective and disease preventative properties and are critical for optimal health.**

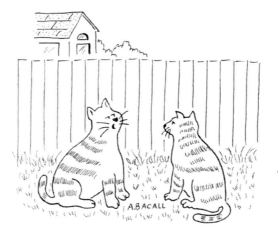

"I take lots of antioxidants. That's why I'm still on the first of my nine lives."

www.cartoonstock.com

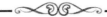

The most important function of antioxidants is to prevent or slow the oxidative damage caused in our bodies by free radicals.

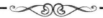

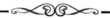 What are free radicals and why should you care about them?

First, the biochemical perspective: Free radicals occur when compounds in a biochemical reaction gain or lose an electron. Missing one or having an uneven number of electrons, the compound becomes oxidized or what we call a free radical—a substance with an unpaired electron. Free radicals are highly reactive and chemically unstable. Mostly they are nasty, removing electrons from stable molecules such as proteins, fatty acids and even DNA. If the loss of electrons is uncontrolled, it can set up a chain reaction which causes excessive oxidation and affects many cells, causing damaging chemical changes in cells.

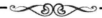

Antioxidants protect us against free radical damage and are critical for optimal health.

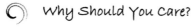

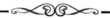 Why Should You Care?

Those chemical changes aren't pretty. **They cause premature aging, wrinkles, arterial damage, inflammation and damage or malfunctioning of DNA which could cause cancer or heart disease.** A certain number of free radicals are however good and our body naturally creates them in certain circumstances.

For example, the metabolism of food and even exercise creates free radicals. This small amount stimulates normal cell growth and division, and destroys infectious agents. **Most people, however, have far too many of them, the result (primarily) of external factors such as industrialization, pollution, smoke, and processed food.**

How do antioxidants protect us from free radicals?

Antioxidants give up electrons to free radicals and therefore neutralize them. The body uses various antioxidants like glutathione, Vitamin A, C and E, beta-carotene, selenium and coenzyme Q10, among others, to neutralize the free radicals.

Antioxidants function best as a team. Two examples of how antioxidants work together are:

- When Vitamin E neutralizes a free radical it becomes a free radical in the process, but Coenzyme Q10, Vitamin C and alpha-lipoic acid turns it back into an antioxidant.
- When Vitamin C recycles Vitamin E, it in turn becomes a free radical, but together alpha-lipoic acid and glutathione convert it back into an antioxidant.

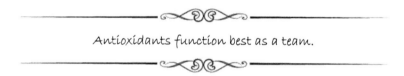

Antioxidants function best as a team.

What are the best sources of antioxidants?

Fruits and vegetables are nature's most abundant source of antioxidants. Nature naturally provides the synergy required for optimal functioning of antioxidants which, as we know, work best in combination with each other.

ORAC (Oxygen Radical Absorbance Capacity)

ORAC is another term you may come across in relation to antioxidants. Simply put, **the ORAC value is a numerical measure indicating the antioxidant capacity or level in a food.**

If a food has a high ORAC value, it has a high antioxidant level, which is, of course, good (since antioxidants neutralize free radicals and decrease our risk of disease). Remember, though: ORAC values are determined in a lab, not in our blood, and therefore only approximate our bodies' ability to absorb and use the antioxidants.

For a comprehensive list, see the following website: www.oracvalues.com/sort/orac-value

The healthiest way to ensure optimum levels of all the micronutrients mentioned so far – vitamins, minerals and antioxidants – is by eating whole foods, particularly legumes, whole grains, fruits and vegetables.

Generally the more colourful the fruits and vegetables, the more nutrients they contain. Foods that are organic, seasonal and/or locally grown generally have a higher concentration of nutrients and are certainly healthier (See Chapter NINE).

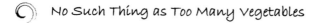

No Such Thing as Too Many Vegetables

If you need any more propagandizing, over the years, researchers have developed a solid base of evidence showing that those who eat a diet high in fruits and vegetables, experience a range of benefits such as:

- Controlling blood pressure.
- Preventing some types of cancer.
- Avoiding diverticulitis (an painful intestinal disease).
- Reducing cataracts and macular degeneration; two common causes of vision loss.

Eating more fruits and veggies also helps you manage weight.

How much should you be eating?

In general; adults should be eating 5-13 servings (2 ½ - 6 ½ cups) of fruit and vegetables every day, depending on your total calorie consumption.

I tell my weight watching clients to limit the number of fruit servings to 1-3, depending on their total nutrient intake per day. **Calorie per nutrient, vegetables come out ahead.**

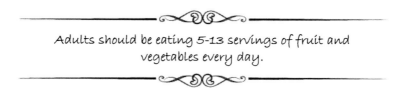

Adults should be eating 5-13 servings of fruit and vegetables every day.

⟲ What makes up a serving?

- 1 cup of raw leafy greens.
- ½ cup cooked or raw vegetables.
- ½ cup fruit.
- ¼ cup dried fruit.

Keep in mind that a cup is about the size of your fist (more on measuring in Chapter SEVEN).

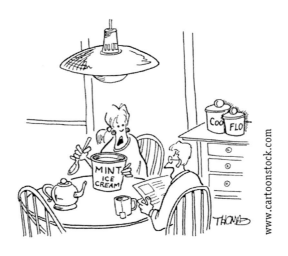

"The doctor told me to introduce more greens in my diet."

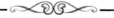

No single fruit or vegetable provides all of the nutrients you need to be healthy so eat different types daily.

Ten Strategies to Make Fruits and Vegetables User-Friendly

1. In following this week's principle, to eat 4-6 nutrient dense meals/snacks each day, make sure each of them includes fruit and/or vegetables.

2. Keep frozen fruits and vegetables for backup.

3. Use frozen fruit instead of ice in smoothies.

4. Buy pre-cut and washed vegetables if it means you'll eat more of them.

5. Wash and cut fresh vegetables and fruit as soon as you get home from shopping to ensure that you have ready-to-eat fresh produce to snack on, add to meals or grab on the run.

6. Always put vegetables on sandwiches (sprouts, avocado and tomato with Swiss cheese; sliced cucumber and red pepper with hummus or Greek salad with green pepper, cucumber, tomato and lettuce stuffed into a pita pocket).

7. Make homemade soups regularly – they're low in calories and sodium, high in nutrients (the secret to great French cooking: throw in all the leftover vegetables).

8. Add extra vegetables to lasagne, casseroles and wherever else they can hide.

9. Keep fruits and vegetables visible and accessible; if you have to take five things out the fridge to get to them, you probably won't eat them.

10. Try a new vegetable and/or fruit each week. Ever try papaya (great for digestion)? Persimmons are honey-sweet; pomegranate seeds – tiny, flavourful rubies.

⟲ WATER

Why is water so important?

- At least 65 percent of your body is water.

- Water is involved in every bodily function.

- Water is a solvent; many substances only become useable when dissolved in water.

- Water is critical in many essential chemical reactions.

- Water transports nutrients and oxygen to cells.

- It eliminates waste and toxins.

- Water is a component of saliva, urine, mucous and, of course, all our blood, sweat and tears.

- **Water helps to "air condition" our bodies.** When we're hot, the hypothalamus portion of our brain receives messages from the temperature receptors in our body signalling the need to cool down. In response, the blood vessels in our skin dilate or grow wide, increasing the flow of blood to our skin. Our sweat glands are then stimulated to produce sweat. Sweat is nothing more than internal heat released into the environment. When we're too cold, the opposite occurs: blood vessels constrict; less blood flows to the skin's surface and less heat is lost through sweating.

- **Water acts as a lubricant**, filling space within and between cells. Without water, our joints would stop moving. We'd stiffen like statues.

- **Water helps regulate our acid-base balance.** We function best when sufficiently alkaline, an environment water sustains (See Chapter NINE).

- **Water is also involved in all metabolic reactions,** including the metabolizing of stored fats, which is one reason it's critical for fat loss and weight management.

How much water do you need to drink?

Generally you should drink about half your body weight (in pounds) in ounces of water. In other words, a person who weighs 140 pounds should drink approximately 70oz. of water per day (about 8-9 glasses). Of course water requirements vary greatly from person to person based body mass, climate, activity level and diet, among other factors. Most importantly, listen to your body and always drink when you are thirsty. However, make sure you are not confusing hunger for thirst (more on that further along).

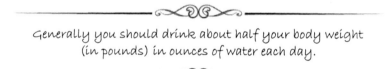

Generally you should drink about half your body weight (in pounds) in ounces of water each day.

During exercise, the American College of Sports Medicine recommends drinking sufficient fluids regularly to avoid a water deficit (as a result of sweating) in excess of 2% body weight.[15] What and when you drink will depend on the duration and intensity of the activity, opportunities to drink, as well as climate.

However be careful not to over hydrate, a condition referred to as hyponatremia that occurs when sodium levels in the blood are diluted due to excessive fluid intake. Although this is a rare condition and is generally only seen in endurance athletes, it can be just as fatal as dehydration which is the more common occurrence in athletes of all levels.

There are two types of dehydration:

- *Acute dehydration* – generally the result of intense physical exercise or illness.

- *Chronic dehydration* – the result of poor hydration over time. Most people are chronically dehydrated, which is often a key explanation for headaches and fatigue.

How do you know if you have either form of dehydration?

For many people, thirst is the first indicator that some degree of dehydration is present.   Other symptoms and changes may include:

- Energy decreases.
- Headaches, dizziness, constipation, dry skin and dry mouth prevail.
- You can't concentrate as well.
- Body temperature rises due to an inability to sweat.
- You're hungry – or think you are.
- Your overall performance declines.
- Metabolism slows.
- Fat burning is compromised.
- Blood and oxygen flow diminishes.
- The heart has to work harder to pump blood.

The point is: don't wait until you are thirsty to hydrate. Get on a regular drinking schedule. Set your watch or phone alarm to ring approximately every 30 minutes as a reminder until you get into the habit. Keep a bottle with you and visible at all times. If you don't see it, chances are you won't remember to use it.

I recommend starting the day with a glass of warm water and lemon – the warm water stimulates the colon and lemon cleanses the liver. Flavouring your water with lemon or fruit slices also makes plain old water a bit more seductive.

Herbal teas are also a good way to bolster your daily intake. Beverages containing alcohol and caffeine, however, are NOT. In fact, both have the opposite effect: they're mild diuretics and tend to dehydrate us. You need extra water when consuming caffeine or alcohol.

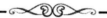

Don't wait until you are thirsty to hydrate.
Get on a regular drinking schedule.

Hungry or Thirsty?

Often when people think they are hungry, their body really wants water. The reason is simple: the sensations for hunger and thirst are generated simultaneously in our brains. We don't recognize the sensations separately and therefore, a person who thinks they are hungry may actually be thirsty (and vice versa although the former is more typical). **The test in either case is simple: drink water. If, a half hour later, you're no longer hungry, chances are you were really thirsty.**

Drinking water before you eat also helps from a weight management perspective. However, you don't want to gulp gallons while you're eating. Too much water while eating dilutes digestive enzymes and therefore compromises digestion. A glass 15 minutes prior to a meal, however, allows enough time for the water to empty out of your stomach. Sipping a small glass with your meal is perfectly acceptable.

Water, water, everywhere, nor any drop to drink."
~The Rime of the Ancient Mariner by Samuel Taylor Coleridge

All waters may be created equal but not necessarily by the time they reach our lips. What type should you drink? The short answer: some type of purified or filtered tap water.

Bottle or Tap?

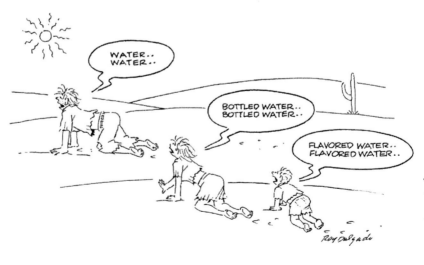

Believe it or not, currently the federal government does not mandate that bottled water be any safer than tap water; the chemical pollution standards are nearly identical. In fact, bottled water is even less regulated than tap water. Close to half of all bottled water is sourced from municipal tap water.

According to the Environmental Working Group, an American non-profit environmental organization, the last label survey (2010) found that the three most basic facts about water namely the source, treatment and purity remained hidden. Overall:

- 18% of bottled waters fail to list the location of their source.
- 32% disclose nothing about the treatment or purity of the water.

Currently the federal government does not mandate that bottled water be any safer than tap water; and close to half of all bottled water is sourced from municipal tap water.

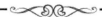

Was their water in fact more pure than tap water?

The report didn't say. And unfortunately, these water quality reports have long since been outdated.

Bottled water is, of course, a convenience. Bear in mind, however, the huge carbon footprint it creates. Every twenty-seven hours, Americans drink enough bottles of water to circle the equator with the empty ones. A more earth-friendly alternative; install some type of water filtration system in your home.[16]

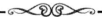

*Every twenty-seven hours, Americans drink enough
bottles of water to circle the equator with the empty ones.*

Buying A Home Water Filter System:

Some questions to think about: Do you want a water filter system that's big or small; budget or deluxe; less or more extensive?

At one end of the spectrum, for example, is a simple Brita® Pitcher with replaceable filters that you can purchase at the local supermarket. At the other end, there are reverse osmosis systems, for example, which will purify the water coming out of every spigot in your house; or you could just install a filter beneath your kitchen sink.

The pitcher system is cheap, and reliable, but it doesn't remove as many contaminants as a reverse osmosis system does. Of course reverse osmosis is more expensive. Other kinds of purification methods (ultra violet filtering, distillation or ion exchange) are available as well. (For more information, go on line or check out www.waterfiltercomparisons.com.)

Whatever type you choose, remember to:
- **Change filters on time.**
- **Carry water in a safe container.** Hard plastic bottles (#7 plastic) can leach a harmful plastics chemical called bisphenol A (BPA) into water. Carry stainless steel or other BPA-free bottles. Don't reuse bottled water bottles; the plastic can harbour bacteria and breakdown to release plastics chemicals.

DIGESTION

> "Happiness: a good bank account, a good
> cook, and a good digestion."
>
> ~Jean-Jacque Rousseau, 18th Century French Philosopher

Nutrients are only half the story; the other half is digestion and absorption. Our body is made of cells, which, of course, are made from the food we eat. **Our bodies – and therefore our cells, are in a constant state of renewal.** For example:

- Skin cells are replaced approximately every 21 days.
- The lining of the digestive tract about every 4 days.
- Red blood cells every 120 days.

In order for these transitions to occur, you need to be able to digest and absorb the food you consume.

The digestive system, and particularly the small intestine, has 2 major functions:

- **To allow useful and necessary substances into the body.**
- **To keep harmful substances out of the body.**

The mechanical process of digestion is performed by chewing our food and from the contraction of muscles along the length of the digestive tract to either move food along or, as in the case of the stomach, to churn food into a softer cool down. The chemical process relies on hormones, enzymes and organs, each of which has a special function.

A quick look at the twin processes of digestion and absorption:

Step One: **You chew.** Saliva emerges. First it helps lubricate the food so you can swallow it. Also, the digestive enzyme, amylase, which is in your saliva, begins digesting carbohydrates.

Step Two: **You swallow.** Aided by peristalsis, the process by which muscles contract, food travels down the esophagus and into the stomach.

Step Three: **Food is soaked in hydrochloric acid and another enzyme, pepsinogen.** When hydrochloric acid and pepsinogen meet, they make pepsin, which begins the process of breaking down protein. Protein is the only nutrient that is partially digested in the stomach.

Note: The stomach can hold about 4 cups of food; more at a given time will compromise the stomach's digestion process. Here is yet another reason to adhere to Principle 5 - Eat Often: 4-6 Meals/Snacks Each Day.

The acidic environment of the stomach helps kill bacteria and viruses. At the same time, enzymes and contracting stomach muscles turn the food into a semi-liquid state known as chyme. Depending on the type, food will remain in the stomach from 30 minutes to four hours.

Step Four: **The stomach releases chyme** into the small intestine in tiny spurts, about a teaspoon size at a time. Here, the rest of the food is digested and absorbed into the bloodstream and lymph vessels. About 90 percent of absorption takes place in the small intestine, whose surface area is huge.

Even the lining of the small intestine requires a high level of nutrients for its maintenance. Food generally remains in the small intestine for three to ten hours. Once absorbed, nutrients are transported through blood and lymph vessels to the various cells of the body.

Your liver, pancreas and gallbladder also aid digestion.

The **liver** serves several functions:

- It produces bile, a substance that helps break down fat and make it more absorbable.
- It metabolizes carbohydrates, protein and fats.
- It stores nutrients.
- It detoxifies drugs and waste products.

The **gallbladder** stores bile and releases it into the small intestine to aid in the absorption of fats. People who've had to have their gallbladders removed have a much harder time absorbing and digesting fat.

The **pancreas** produces and secretes enzymes such as protease to break down protein; lipase to break down fats, and amylase to break down carbohydrates. It also produces and secretes the hormone insulin to aid in the absorption of glucose.

Step Five: Once all this occurs, that which remains of the eaten food – **water and waste – moves into the large intestines.** There, it is "attacked" by various bacterial strains that reside in the colon. Their action causes water to be reabsorbed and stool made. Waste generally remains in the colon for 24-72 hours. A slow transit time of waste out of the colon allows toxins to be reabsorbed, which increases the risk of certain diseases; hence, the stress on eating enough and water to insure regularity.

When all goes well, the digestive process keeps you in optimal health. **Here are some simple steps you can take to improve your digestion:**

1. Eat slowly and chew food thoroughly.
2. Do not eat when you are stressed (See Chapter THREE).
3. Do not overeat (your stomach can only comfortably hold 4 cups maximum at any time).
4. Do not drink too much fluid with meals.

If digestion is still a problem, you may want to try either of these additional techniques:

Food combining: of which the basic premise is to essentially eat protein, starchy carbohydrates and fats separately. For example, good food combining would be a meal of animal protein and non-starchy vegetables or, starchy foods/grains with vegetables.

According to the food combining theory, fats go best with non-starchy vegetables; second best with grains and avoid combining with proteins. Fruit should be eaten alone and on an empty stomach – either 30 minutes before meals or at least two hours after a meal.

Digestive enzymes; these are available over the counter. For a more complete discussion on supplements, see Chapter NINE.

Putting It All Together

Principle 5 - Eat Often: 4-6 Nutrient Dense Meals/Snacks Each Day

As discussed previously, going without eating for long periods (typically more than three hours), causes blood sugar levels to dip. Your body will tell you (via cravings) that you need sugar and you need it quickly. At this point, you'll probably head straight for the vending machine or nearest Starbucks® or coffee shop for a quick sugar fix – a donut, a muffin, a chocolate bar or one of those deceptively "light chinos". Despite the best of intentions, when blood sugar levels drop, sugar is what you will crave. And your body, in its wisdom, knows a chicken breast just won't cut it. Fruit is, of course, a better option than a donut, but why put yourself in this precarious position at all?

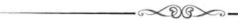

Going without eating for long periods (typically more than three hours), causes blood sugar levels to dip, when blood sugar levels drop, sugar is what you will crave.

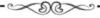

Eating every couple of hours is one way to avoid leaving yourself vulnerable to the sugar-cravings. However, what you eat during those intervals matters too. Sugary, processed foods will very soon put you back into the same position. Balanced, nutrient dense meals, on the other hand, will lessen your cravings, sustain your energy and stabilize your mood. And isn't that good news?

A Sample of My Favourite Healthy Meals and Snacks

Top Three Breakfasts:

- Protein smoothie (whey protein powder, Greek yogurt, almond milk and frozen berries with some ground flaxseeds or flaxseed oil).

- Protein pancakes (40g uncooked oatmeal, ½ cup of egg whites with a couple tablespoons of ground flaxseed) served with berries or a banana and sometimes a little almond butter.

- Two scrambled eggs with grilled tomato and mushrooms and Ezekiel toast.

Top Lunch and Dinner Options (Mine are always quick, easy to prepare and transportable):

- Baked sweet potato, tuna mixed with salsa and cut up vegetables or a spinach salad with flaxseed oil dressing.

- Lean steak in a vegetable stir fry with brown rice.

- Grilled salmon with quinoa and grilled vegetables.

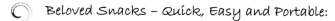

Beloved Snacks – Quick, Easy and Portable:

- Apple with either a tablespoon of almond butter or two Babybel® cheese.
- Cut up vegetables (peppers and cucumber) with hummus or ricotta cheese.
- Pineapple with ricotta cheese.
- Vega Vibrancy Bar© or Lara Bar©.
- Greek yogurt with flaxseed, ½ a banana, drop of unpasteurized honey.
- Babybel® cheese and almonds.

For some people, the fewer choices and lesser variety – the easier it is to stay on track. Also, you spend less time thinking about food, which is especially liberating for the chronic dieter. Consider having the same two options for lunch and dinner for a month, or the same morning and afternoon snack for a month; then shake things up a bit. Again, your strategy will depend on your personality – the "less variety" approach works best for busy people who don't have much time to think or prepare.

Whatever your strategy:

- **Have healthy foods prepared and ready to go** (more in Chapter SEVEN).

- **Never leave home without a couple of snacks**, even if running out for a quick errand. You never know how your day can change.

- **Plan the timing of your meals within your schedule.** For example, if I'm eating breakfast at 7a.m. and have a lunch date at 1p.m., I'll make sure to have a small snack mid-morning. If on the other hand, lunch is scheduled for noon and I eat breakfast at 9a.m., I'll skip the snack; maybe save it for later in the afternoon. Forewarned, you can be forearmed.

Change4Good Nutrition GPS©

You now know the basics – and more – about nutrition. **Next step: assess where your habits need improvements most urgently.** You set up a Change4Good Attitude and Behaviour GPS©. Now do one for nutrition.

 Checkpoints: **You'll notice these largely conform to the 10 Change4Good Principles,** some of which are laid out in more detail in future chapters. In the meantime, it's wise to consider issues like portion control, label-reading and moderation anyway.

- **Protein** – lean and includes plant sources?
- **Carbohydrates** – natural or processed and refined?
- **Fats** – healthy and daily? Do you (mostly) avoid saturated, hydrogenated and trans fats?
- **Water** – drink 1-2 litres a day?
- **Fruits** – do you eat 1-3 servings of fruit per day?
- **Vegetables** – At least 4-6 servings daily?
- **Timing** – healthy meal or snack roughly every 3 hours?
- **Combo platter** – do you combine lean protein, natural carbohydrates and healthy fats at every meal?
- **Journal** – is all that you consume written in it faithfully?
- **Sleuth** – do you read food labels like a pro?
- **New Math** – do you monitor portions?
- **90/10** – splurge but demurely?

As before, **below is an example of a completed Change4Good Nutrition GPS©** as well as a blank one for you to complete. If you prefer, you can download a copy at **www.change4good.ca.**

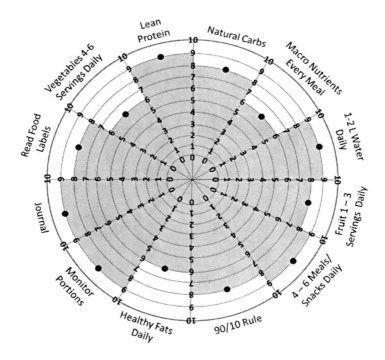

Change Your Nutrition

What to do:

1. Using the Change4Good Nutrition GPS© rate your level of satisfaction for each separate area between zero and ten (ten being complete satisfaction; zero being none).

2. Place one dot (per segment) opposite the number that best represents your level of satisfaction.

3. Connect the dots to create a "circle" within the Change4Good Nutrition GPS©. **Unless you're consistently compliant, the circle-within-the-circle is bound to be** *asymmetrical.*

Eat Often: 4-6 Nutrient-Dense Meals/Snacks Each Day

Your Change4Good Nutrition GPS©

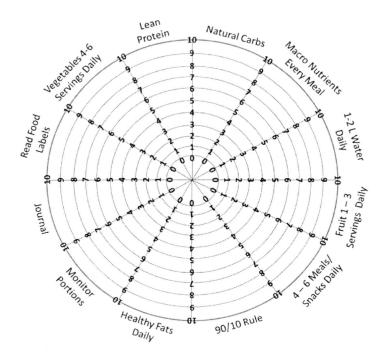

Now, again, consider the following:

1. **How large is your circle?** Bigger is better.
2. **How symmetrical is it?** Your goal is to push everything to the outer rim, to have the largest, roundest circle.
3. **Where does your circle dip toward the center? The dips indicate the areas you most need to address.** Keep them in mind as you complete your Change4Good action steps.

CHANGE4GOOD – ACTION STEPS

- Start implementing Principle 5 - Eat Often: 4-6 Nutrient Dense Meals/Snacks Each Day.

- Complete your Change4Good Nutrition GPS©.

- Identify and complete your fourth Short - Term (Weekly) Goal. Your Nutrition GPS should help. For example: "I will always keep a healthy snack with me, no matter where I go; I will keep a filled water bottle in my car. I'll add new fruits and vegetables (pomegranate seeds, papaya and kabocha squash – tastes like pumpkin pie)."

- Update Change4Good Journal© daily.

- Update Change4Good Goal Sheet© weekly.

TOOLS

- Change4Good Goal Sheet©

- Change4Good Journal©

- Change4Good Nutrition GPS©

REMEMBER THIS

- G-d is in the details, also in micronutrients.

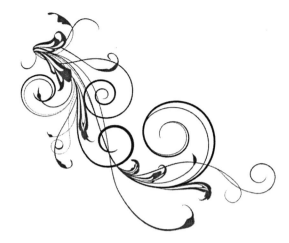

Chapter SIX

Change Your Nutrition

OUR KITCHENS/OURSELVES— DEMYSTIFYING FOOD LABELS

This chapter is about hacking your way through the labels jungle, and filling your fridge with foods that you love – and that will love you back.

Principle 6 Read: Those Tricky Food Labels

Through advertising, food companies try to lure you into buying the wrong stuff. Usually they succeed. Not anymore. Learn to read labels (and the fine print) like a pro.

"If you can organize your kitchen, you can organize your life."

~Louis Parrish, M.D., Author

Would you buy a book without at least reading the jacket; or a television without studying its features, of course not. **Yet you probably toss bags and boxes into your shopping cart without really knowing what's in them.** "Low fat!" a box of children's cereal screams. And yet the cereal is loaded with enough sugar to vanquish its healthful other claims. "No preservatives", another shouts. But what about all the dyes used to color those little marshmallows?

This chapter teaches you how to shop smart. Armed with the knowledge of what to buy, you'll be ready to create a dream kitchen – not in terms of décor but in terms of how beautifully it will furbish your insides.

The Labels Jungle

Nutrition Facts

Serving Size 2 oz. (56.7g)

Servings per Container	1	
Calories 210	Calories from Fat 60	
		%DV
Total Fat 6g		9%
Saturated Fat 1.5g		8%
Trans Fat 0g		
Cholesterol 0mg		0%
Sodium 180mg		8%
Potassium 200mg		6%
Total Carbohydrate 25g		8%
Dietary Fibre 4g		16%
Sugars 13g		
Protein 18g		8%

Vitamin A 0%	Vitamin C 2%	Calcium 6%
Phosphorus 20%	Magnesium 10%	Iron 20%

Percent Daily Values (DV) are based on a 2,000 calorie diet. Your daily values may be higher or lower depending on your calorie needs.

		Calories	2000	2500
Total Fat	Less than		65g	80g
Saturated Fat	Less than		20g	30g
Cholesterol	Less than		300mg	300mg
Sodium	Less than		2,400mg	2,400mg
Total Carbohydrate			300g	375g
Dietary Fibre			25g	30g

Granted your local supermarket isn't a museum; you aren't there to spend all day studying *objets d'art* at close range. Still, it pays to spend some time learning to decipher labels.

Two items are of importance:

- **The Nutrition Facts Table** (which gives the amounts of calories, servings and nutrients).
- **The list of ingredients**, which tells you exactly what's in what you're eating.

Below, is what you should look for on a label:

◔ Understanding Food Labels

1. SERVING SIZE:

Serving size, by definition is the standard amount of food recommended for a particular food/nutrient.

A serving size of your favourite muffin may only be 150 calories, but it's also only half a muffin. And are you really going to eat only a half? The moral of the story: check what the manufacturer considers a serving size. Also, notice all the information on the Nutrition Facts Label is calibrated per serving size.

Nutrition Facts		
Serving Size 2 oz. (56.7g)		
Servings per Container	1	
Calories 210	Calories from Fat 60	
		%DV
Total Fat 6g		9%
Saturated Fat 1.5g		8%
Trans Fat 0g		
Cholesterol 0mg		0%
Sodium 180mg		8%
Potassium 200mg		6%
Total Carbohydrate 25g		8%
Dietary Fibre 4g		16%
Sugars 13g		
Protein 18g		8%
Vitamin A 0%	Vitamin C 2%	Calcium 6%
Phosphorus 20%	Magnesium 10%	Iron 20%

Percent Daily Values (DV) are based on a 2,000 calorie diet. Your daily values may be higher or lower depending on your calorie needs.			
	Calories	2000	2500
Total Fat	Less than	65g	80g
Saturated Fat	Less than	20g	30g
Cholesterol	Less than	300mg	300mg
Sodium	Less than	2,400mg	2,400mg
Total Carbohydrate		300g	375g
Dietary Fibre		25g	30g

The serving size of this item is 2 oz. (56.7g), and there is one serving in the container.

2. CALORIES PER SERVING SIZE:

When you marry serving size with calories per serving size, boy do you get surprises.

Recently, I challenged a friend who considered cold cereal a reasonably virtuous snack to pour herself a bowl. An avalanche of cereal flowed into her bowl. "Now see how many servings you're actually eating?" Although the calories per serving size on the label were a reasonable 110, my friend, consuming 3 serving sizes, was consuming 330 calories (not counting the skim milk she poured into her bowl).

Once you compare serving size with calories per serving size, you'll probably change your choice of post-dinner snacks or at least reduce the quantity. Plain oatmeal, for example, also has approximately 110 calories for a single serving, and cooked in water, it delivers a reasonable half bowl.

Nutrition Facts		
Serving Size 2 oz. (56.7g)		
Servings per Container		1
Calories 210		Calories from Fat 60
		%DV
Total Fat 6g		9%
Saturated Fat 1.5g		8%
Trans Fat 0g		
Cholesterol 0mg		0%
Sodium 180mg		8%
Potassium 200mg		6%
Total Carbohydrate 25g		8%
Dietary Fibre 4g		16%
Sugars 13g		
Protein 18g		8%
Vitamin A 0%	Vitamin C 2%	Calcium 6%
Phosphorus 20%	Magnesium 10%	Iron 20%

Percent Daily Values (DV) are based on a 2,000 calorie diet. Your daily values may be higher or lower depending on your calorie needs.			
	Calories	2000	2500
Total Fat	Less than	65g	80g
Saturated Fat	Less than	20g	30g
Cholesterol	Less than	300mg	300mg
Sodium	Less than	2,400mg	2,400mg
Total Carbohydrate		300g	375g
Dietary Fibre		25g	30g

This item has 210 calories per serving and there is 1 serving in the container.

The point; do the math and take calories and serving size seriously. **A snack should be between 100-200 calories, and a meal** (depending on your goal and body weight) **should be between 300–500 calories.**

3. TOTAL CARBOHYDRATES:

This unit of measurement consists of the sum of dietary fibre and sugars, sugar alcohols and starch. (The latter two, even if present, are not always listed).

Nutrition Facts	
Serving Size 2 oz. (56.7g)	
Servings per Container	1
Calories 210	Calories from Fat 60
	%DV
Total Fat 6g	9%
Saturated Fat 1.5g	8%
Trans Fat 0g	
Cholesterol 0mg	0%
Sodium 180mg	8%
Potassium 200mg	6%
Total Carbohydrate 25g	8%
Dietary Fibre 4g	16%
Sugars 13g	
Protein 18g	8%

	Vitamin C 2%	Calcium 6%
Phosphorus 20%	Magnesium 10%	Iron 20%

Percent Daily Values (DV) are based on a 2,000 calorie diet. Your daily values may be higher or lower depending on your calorie needs.			
	Calories	2000	2500
Total Fat	Less than	65g	80g
Saturated Fat	Less than	20g	30g
Cholesterol	Less than	300mg	300mg
Sodium	Less than	2,400mg	2,400mg
Total Carbohydrate		300g	375g
Dietary Fibre		25g	30g

One serving of carbohydrate is 15 grams.

Typically, you consume more than one serving when you eat a portion of food.

This item has 25 grams of total carbohydrate, which is just less than 2 servings of carbohydrate.

Let's break these components down:

- Dietary Fibre – the higher the fibre amount, the more slowly the food will be absorbed into the bloodstream and the lower your insulin response. **Ideally, look for products with 4 grams or more of fibre per serving.**

- Sugars – **if more than one sugar source appears in the first 3-5 ingredients, think twice about buying the item.** The ingredients will tell you if the sugars are natural, added or artificial. Consider the trillion types of sugar: brown sugar, cane sugar, corn syrup, dextrin, evaporated cane juice, fruit juice concentrate, high fructose corn syrup, honey, invert sugar, malt, maple syrup, molasses, raw sugar, turbinado sugar, grape juice, sucrose, dextrose, maltose, lactose, mannitol, sorbitol and on and on.

If more than one sugar source appears in the first 3-5 ingredients, think twice about buying the item.

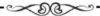

A teaspoon of granulated table sugar is approximately 4-5 grams. In terms of calories, all sugars may be the same; in terms of nutrients and glycemic value, they are not. For example, regardless of whether I'm eating a chocolate bar or an apple, I'm eating sugar and possibly the same amount. However, an apple has fructose and fibre, both of which help slow down its digestion. Any factor that slows digestion helps minimize the amount of insulin released.

In addition, apples have water, vitamins, minerals and antioxidants – all adding to our body's nutrient stores. Chocolate however, requires the use of our stored nutrients in order to be digested and absorbed. Apples nourish and chocolate depletes – one of many reasons apples, or any other natural whole food, are always the better nutritional bet.

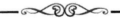

Any factor that slows digestion helps minimize the amount of insulin released.

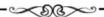

- *Starch* – In numerical terms, it's the difference between the total number of carbohydrates, on the one hand, and the sum of the grams of sugar and fibre on the other. For example, a serving of Kashi Go Lean® (see next page) contains 37 grams of total carbohydrates – which are the sum of the 5 grams of fibre, 9 grams of sugar and 23 grams of starch. In terms of composition, starch is a complex sugar and is digested more slowly.

Ideally, then, you want the amount of sugar to be low, and the fibre and starch to be higher relative to the sugar. By law, starch does not have to be listed on labels. Two examples:

Kashi Go Lean® Cereal

1 cup (55g)
37g of Total Carbohydrate (approximately 2 servings
        of carbohydrate)
5g Fibre
9g Sugar
23g Starch (it is, in fact, listed on the label).

Shasha Organic® Spelt bread

2 slices (64 g)
30g of Total Carbohydrate (2 servings of carbohydrate)
3g of Fibre
2g of Sugar
The balance of 25g (not listed but 30g minus 5g) would be starch.

A tip when buying cereals, besides considering the ingredients (more on that to follow); **look for cereals with less than 2 grams of fat, more than 3 grams of fibre and less than 8 grams of sugar per 100 calories.**

*Ideally, then, you want the amount of sugar to be low,
and the fibre and starch to be higher relative to the sugar.*

- *Sugar Alcohols* - As discussed in Chapter FOUR, these are mostly only found in *so-called low-carbohydrate products*. When sugar alcohols are used in a product, the total amount of carbohydrate is described as **Net Carbs.**

Net Carbs is a term that refers to the amount of carbohydrates that will affect blood glucose, and therefore insulin levels. The term arose in the wake of high-protein diets (Atkins®, and the like), which advocated the use of sugar alcohols as a way to sweeten foods without causing a spike in blood sugar and insulin levels. **Note: I don't generally recommend the kind of processed foods in which sugar alcohols appear.**

4. PROTEIN: **30 grams equals one serving of protein.**

   This item has 18 grams of protein which is just more than half a protein serving.

   See Chapter FOUR for the average amount of protein people need, relative to their lifestyle, size, gender and other factors.

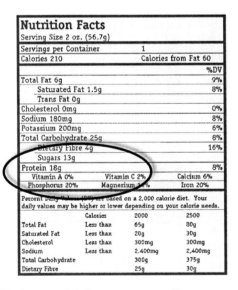

Animal products generally have a higher amount of protein per serving-size than plant proteins.

For example, you'd need nearly three servings of beans to get the same amount of protein per single serving of turkey or chicken. **Always choose lean proteins.**

5. FATS: These are trickier to calculate. **5 grams equals one serving of fat.** First, check out the total amount of fat per serving.

   This item has 6 grams and 60 calories of total fat per serving.

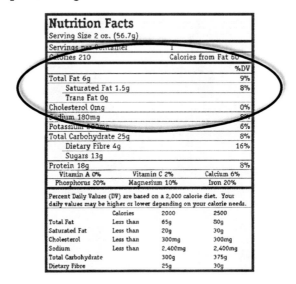

To determine the percentage of fat in a serving:

- Divide the calories from fat (60) by the total number of calories in the serving (210).
- Then multiply by 100.

For example: 60/210 = .29. Multiply by 100 to get 29. That means **29% of this item's calories come from fat.**

In general, you want to avoid foods whose fat contents are more than 20%-35% of the total calories in the food; more simply stay under 2–3.5 grams or 20-35 calories of fat per 100 calories.

6. *QUALITY OF FATS:* As important as the quantity is the
    quality of the fat.

    **Avoid any hydrogenated or partially hydrogenated fats
    and oils, and trans-fats or oils.** These fats, the
    unhealthiest fats of all, lead to heart disease and cancer;
    shun any and all. As for cholesterol, don't have more
    than 300 mg a day. (One egg contains 200 mg of
    cholesterol, all of it in the yolk).

**Saturated fats should be
limited; no more than
10 percent of a person's
total fat intake** should
be from saturated fats.

**This item has 1.5 grams
of saturated fat
per serving and 0 grams
of trans-fats.**

**Good quality fats
include the
monounsaturated and
polyunsaturated fats.**
Even people

Nutrition Facts		
Serving Size 2 oz. (56.7g)		
Servings per Container	1	
Calories 210	Calories from Fat 60	
		%DV
Total Fat 6g		9%
Saturated Fat 1.5g		8%
Trans Fat 0g		
Cholesterol 0mg		0%
Sodium 180mg		7%
Potassium 280mg		6%
Total Carbohydrate 25g		8%
Dietary Fibre 4g		16%
Sugars 13g		
Protein 18g		8%
Vitamin A 0%	Vitamin C 2%	Calcium 6%
Phosphorus 20%	Magnesium 10%	Iron 20%

Percent Daily Values (DV) are based on a 2,000 calorie diet. Your daily values may be higher or lower depending on your calorie needs.			
	Calories	2000	2500
Total Fat	Less than	65g	80g
Saturated Fat	Less than	20g	30g
Cholesterol	Less than	300mg	300mg
Sodium	Less than	2,400mg	2,400mg
Total Carbohydrate		300g	375g
Dietary Fibre		25g	30g

maintaining a healthy weight shouldn't have more than
35 percent of their calories come from fat.

Remember, as we saw in Chapter FOUR, fat is important
to overall good health, which is why I'd steer clear of
fat-free diets unless your doctor insists.

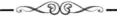

*Avoid any hydrogenated or partially hydrogenated fats and
oils, and trans-fats or oils. Saturated fats should be limited;
no more than 10 percent of a person's total fat intake.*

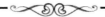

7. SODIUM: You'd be amazed at how much salt frozen, canned and pre-packaged foods contain – even (and sometimes especially) so-called healthy foods like vegetarian soups or burgers.

In general, don't consume more than 1500-2300mg of sodium a day (which, believe it or not, is only 1 teaspoon).

This item has 180mg of sodium per serving.

For frozen meals, buy those with less than 400mg of sodium for the entire meal.

Nutrition Facts		
Serving Size 2 oz. (56.7g)		
Servings per Container	1	
Calories 210		Calories from Fat 60
		%DV
Total Fat 6g		9%
Saturated Fat 1.5g		8%
Trans Fat 0g		
Cholesterol 0mg		0%
Sodium 180mg		8%
Potassium 200mg		6%
Total Carbohydrate 25g		8%
Dietary Fibre 4g		16%
Sugars 13g		
Protein 18g		8%
Vitamin A 0%	Vitamin C 2%	Calcium 6%
Phosphorus 20%	Magnesium 10%	Iron 20%

Percent Daily Values (DV) are based on a 2,000 calorie diet. Your daily values may be higher or lower depending on your calorie needs.			
	Calories	2000	2500
Total Fat	Less than	65g	80g
Saturated Fat	Less than	20g	30g
Cholesterol	Less than	300mg	300mg
Sodium	Less than	2,400mg	2,400mg
Total Carbohydrate		300g	375g
Dietary Fibre		25g	30g

In general, the less sodium in any packaged food, the better. Better to do your salting yourself and avoid salted or processed foods.

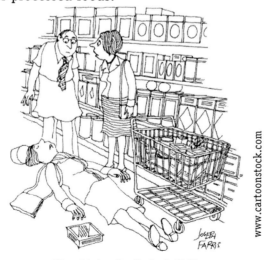

"She read the ingredients listed on the label!"

www.cartoonstock.com

Read: Those Tricky Food Labels

8. PERCENTAGE DAILY VALUE: **The % Daily Values (%DVs) tells you what percent of a particular nutrient is in a single-serving size of a particular food.**

The percentages are based on general recommendations established by the government of how much of a key nutrient you should eat each day; assuming a 2,000 calorie daily diet.

The %DV lets you know if a serving of food is high or low in a particular nutrient. For example 5%DV or less is considered low. 20%DV or more is considered high.

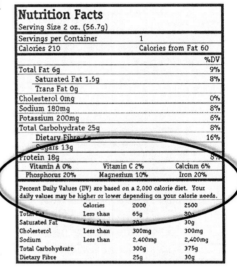

Nutrition Facts

Serving Size 2 oz. (56.7g)		
Servings per Container	1	
Calories 210	Calories from Fat 60	

		%DV
Total Fat 6g		9%
Saturated Fat 1.5g		8%
Trans Fat 0g		
Cholesterol 0mg		0%
Sodium 180mg		8%
Potassium 200mg		6%
Total Carbohydrate 25g		8%
Dietary Fibre 4g		16%
Sugars 13g		
Protein 18g		8%

Vitamin A 0%	Vitamin C 2%	Calcium 6%
Phosphorus 20%	Magnesium 10%	Iron 20%

Percent Daily Values (DV) are based on a 2,000 calorie diet. Your daily values may be higher or lower depending on your calorie needs.

		Calories	2000	2500
Total Fat	Less than		65g	80g
Saturated Fat	Less than		20g	30g
Cholesterol	Less than		300mg	300mg
Sodium	Less than		2,400mg	2,400mg
Total Carbohydrate			300g	375g
Dietary Fibre			25g	30g

For example, this item contains 2%DV of Vitamin C, which is considered low, but 20%DV of iron, which is considered high.

Note: Most labels include recommended %DV for the following:

- Total fat and saturated fat (excluding trans fats).
- Sodium.
- Total carbohydrate and fibre.
- Vitamin A, Vitamin C, calcium and iron.

They do not typically list a %DV for protein since most people get enough, and they do not typically list %DV for sugar because there is no generally accepted "required" amount of sugar for a healthy population. The listing of %DV for cholesterol is optional.

The %DV is helpful because it allows you to quickly distinguish one abstract nutrient claim from another, such as "reduced fat" vs. "light" or "non-fat". Just compare the %DVs for total fat in each food product to see which one is higher or lower in that nutrient.

9. ORDER OF INGREDIENTS: Elsewhere on the package (and sometimes you really have to look) are the list of ingredients.

Here, ingredients are listed in descending order by weight, i.e., the ingredient that weighs the most is listed first.

Ingredients that make up less than 2% of the food by weight are listed at the end or not at all. These ingredients may include flavour enhancers, stabilizers, or other such agents. The ingredients list will also inform you amply about the nutritional quality of a product.

Sample Ingredient Listing from a meal replacement bar:

INGREDIENTS: Soy protein isolate, Energy Blend (fructose, natural extract of chicory, dextrose), ground almonds, brown rice syrup, Energy Smart™ (fruit juice, natural grain dextrins) soy crisps (soy protein isolate, rice flour, calcium carbonate), soy nuts, cocoa powder, agave nectar, textured soy flour, chocolate liquor, natural flavours, fructose, salt, inulin.

> Ideally, the fewer ingredients, the better. Beware of long
> lists of ingredients you don't recognize. In general: if you
> do not recognize many ingredients, don't buy the item.

10. MARKETING STRATEGIES:

**For the most accurate information about the product,
skip the claims on the package and head straight for the
nutrition facts panel and ingredients list.** Just to show
you how much the hype on the package differs from the
actual nutritional contents of the food, examine the label
of a healthy-sounding item – a well-known brand of a
popular cereal bar. Look at all the lovely qualities about
which the manufacturer boasts on the package:

"8g whole grains...."
"One good decision can lead to another..."
"Antioxidants rich in Vitamin C and E"

Now look at the actual ingredients; are these the
substances you'd want to put into your body?

INGREDIENTS: CRUST: WHOLE GRAIN OATS, WHOLE WHEAT FLOUR,
ENRICHED FLOUR (WHEAT FLOUR, NIACIN, REDUCED IRON, THIAMIN
MONONITRATE [VITAMIN B1], RIBOFLAVIN [VITAMIN B2], FOLIC ACID),
SUGAR, SOYBEAN OIL WITH TBHQ FOR FRESHNESS, SOLUBLE CORN FIBRE,
WHEAT BRAN, CALCIUM CARBONATE, DEXTROSE, SALT, CELLULOSE,
POTASSIUM BICARBONATE, MONO- AND DIGLYCERIDES, ASCORBIC ACID
(VITAMIN C), ALPHA TOCOPHEROL ACETATE (VITAMIN E), SOY LECITHIN,
NATURAL AND ARTIFICIAL FLAVOR, WHEAT GLUTEN, CORNSTARCH, NONFAT
MILK, NIACINAMIDE, VITAMIN A PALMITATE, CARRAGEENAN, ZINC OXIDE,
REDUCED IRON, GUAR GUM, PYRIDOXINE HYDROCHLORIDE (VITAMIN B6),
THIAMIN HYDROCHLORIDE (VITAMIN B1), RIBOFLAVIN (VITAMIN B2), FOLIC
ACID). FILLING: INVERT SUGAR, CORN SYRUP, WATER, GLYCERIN, CHERRY
PUREE CONCENTRATE, SUGAR, MODIFIED CORN STARCH, POMEGRANATE JUICE
CONCENTRATE, SODIUM ALGINATE, SODIUM CITRATE, NATURAL AND
ARTIFICIAL FLAVOR, MALIC ACID, CITRIC ACID, METHYLCELLULOSE,
DICALCIUM PHOSPHATE, CARAMEL COLOR, RED #40.

Below are some points to consider regarding marketing strategies:

1. Know the legal definitions for the most common nutrient content claims:

Sugar:	Sugar free:	The product provides less than 0.5 grams per serving.
	Reduced sugar:	The food contains at least 25% less sugar per serving than the reference food.
Calories:	Calorie free:	The food provides fewer than 5 kcal per serving.
	Low calorie:	The food provides 40 kcal or less per serving.
	Reduced calories:	The food contains at least 25% fewer kcal per serving than the reference food.
Fat:	Fat free:	The food provides less than 0.5 grams of fat per serving.
	Low fat:	The food contains 3 grams or less of fat per serving.
	Reduced fat:	The food supplies at least 25% less fat per serving than the reference food – but of course that could still be huge, depending on the food.
Cholesterol:	Cholesterol free:	The food contains less than 2mg of cholesterol and 2 grams or less of saturated fat per serving.
Fibre:	High source of fibre:	The food contains 4 grams or more of per serving.
	Source of fibre:	The food supplies 2 grams or more of fibre per serving (Note: you'd have to eat 15 servings to get a decent amount of fibre).
Meat and Poultry:	Extra lean:	The food contains 7.5% or less fat.
	Lean:	The food contains 10% or less fat (Note: Either lean or extra lean, a meat product can still contain a significant amount of fat).

Read: Those Tricky Food Labels

2. Know the meaning of these often misinterpreted terms:

Enriched:	Food processing often depletes the food of its natural nutrient supply. To compensate, the manufacturer adds back some of what was lost. Hence, the food is called "enriched." Ironically, the so-called "enriched" item usually has fewer nutrients than the original, unprocessed and un-enriched item - not the way most people would interpret the term "enriched."
Fortified:	Additional nutrients that weren't originally in the food are added. Often, the quantity is not really enough to have any significant impact on health; yet, you'll probably be charged more for this item.

3. Deconstruct the meaning of health organization logos on packaging:

The name or logo of a particular non-profit health organization on a package probably leads you to believe that that product must be healthy. Why else would the organization endorse it? Wrong.

In many cases, the label is there as part of a *quid pro quo*: the manufacturer asks the health organization if it can use its logo. The health organization may say yes but not without strings. Manufacturers usually pay huge amounts of money to these organizations for the privilege of using their logos, knowing they may entice you to purchase the product.

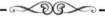

Skip the hype or even the endorsements and turn straight to the nutrition panel and list of ingredients.

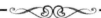

4. The whole truth?

Food manufactures can't put false information on a product, but they can mislead you. For example, a company may put "no cholesterol" on a box of dried fruit. Of course dried fruit doesn't have cholesterol. Still, by putting it on the label, the manufacturer is banking on your willingness to spend more for what you think is the unique absence of cholesterol in this particular brand. **Be very hip: avoid hype.**

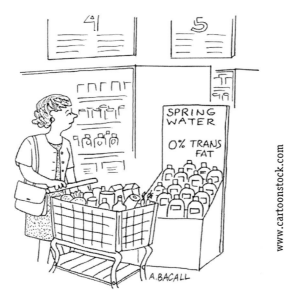

5. Don't be fooled by graphics

A particular brand of cereal pictures a cyclist on the box. "Oh, this must be a healthy cereal," you think. Wrong. The cereal in question is loaded with sugar and possibly other ingredients that are useless in terms of health. **Remember: food manufacturers don't only try to fool kids.**

YOUR DREAM KITCHEN

And I don't mean tiles and ceiling fixtures. I mean what's inside those beautiful cabinets and cupboards and even outside, on your counters, in your refrigerator and on your shelves. Nothing makes a kitchen look worse than boxes of processed foods scattered everywhere. But fill a gorgeous ceramic bowl with shiny green apples – now that's an accessory that never goes out of style.

So, where to begin? Flip on some music, turn up your iPod and start cleaning. Obviously, you can't throw out the items that other people in your house (children, spouse, partner) prefer (at least not yet), but notice how the more healthy foods you stock (and display attractively), the more healthy foods everyone starts to eat. **Keep the healthy foods visible and accessible.** We're talking about your kitchen here, but the same ideas apply to your office and any other environment in which you may store food.

A word on breaking up with old lovers (or How To Throw Out Ice Cream). It's almost impossible for a person to pull out a bag of frozen organic broccoli when three pints of Ben & Jerry's® are in open view. In that case, your environment is easy to fix. Hide the ice cream (or throw it out). Impossible, I know. Better not to have it around in the first place. If I want a treat, and sometimes, often, I do, I find it better to set up my life so that I have go out to get it. Amazing how my craving for chocolate dissipates when I have to step out into the chill February air to indulge it. The same goes for your non-food environment, too (Chapter THREE). If you loathe your job, aren't happy in your relationship, find yourself lethargic and uninspired, then more than just your food needs changing. Eating and living, as I've said, go hand in hand. The funny thing is that small changes like improving your overall physical health and wellbeing can lead to other changes, both in your mental, emotional and even spiritual life.

To affirm the above: **it is well known that just seeing tempting foods provokes hunger.** It also causes the release of dopamine, a brain chemical that produces a feel-good sensation and may intensify a particular craving. **Put trigger foods in opaque containers and if you must keep them, stow them where they aren't visible.**

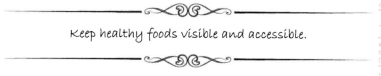

Keep healthy foods visible and accessible.

De-clutter: the heart and soul of most homes is the kitchen which often becomes a railway station crowded with non-food related activity and mess.

For some, clutter leads to stress, which raises cortisol levels in the blood – which, of course, increases hunger. Try, instead:

- To use the kitchen for cooking and eating only.

- Keep the mail, newspapers and keys in their designated places.

- Keep your counters clear so you can use them for chopping vegetables or displaying healthy snacks like a rainbow-assortment of crudités or whatever fruits and herbs or plants looked great at the market that day.

Between meals, keep the lights off in the kitchen – a subtle hint that says the kitchen is closed. Make another room the gathering spot for recreation.

Read: *Those Tricky Food Labels*

The Art of Eating Peaceably

Your dream kitchen is the place where you and your family go to nourish not just your body but your self. How appropriate, then, to eat in a manner that shows respect for your body and its needs. What I'm saying is that given all that food does for our bodies, eating is practically holy. Revere it. Eat consciously and without distractions (see Change4Good Principle 1).

Brian Wansink confirms through various studies that people who eat while watching television, working or being otherwise distracted, consume at least 15%, but as high as 40% more food and eat more frequently[17]. But if all you do while you eat is eat; you're much more likely to listen to hunger cues and enjoy the act of heeding them. You can't always avoid eating on the run or hastily – but try.

PLANNING, LISTING, SHOPPING

 Phase I: MEAL PLANNING

How many times have you come home, walked into the kitchen, stared into the fridge and stressed about what to make for dinner – then realized you didn't have the ingredients for what you finally decided you did want to make? Or even worse, because of all the above, ordered in or picked up pizza – again? **By setting aside 10-15 minutes each week you can avoid the "What's for dinner?" syndrome.**

Note: eating junk food or convenience food requires no planning. But following the Change4Good Principles© – losing weight or successfully maintaining a healthy weight – does.

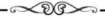

By setting aside 10-15 minutes each week you can avoid the "What's for dinner?" syndrome.

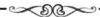

Get used to it. And once you do, you'll find it all surprisingly easy, a habit, like learning how to ski or put on eyeliner or throw a curve ball. During your commute or while on your treadmill plan what you will have each night. Keep quicker, simpler meals for your long or busy days.

Addendum: Plan not only what you will eat – plan when you will eat it too. It provides security and freedom from needless thinking about food. Then move on to Phase II.

Phase II: GROCERY LIST

A present: a general grocery list to download and use as a guide (www.change4good.ca). Where possible, I've listed specific brand products; check the labels yourself, however, and make sure the products suit your Nutrition GPS.

Remember: frozen are as good, if not better than fresh, and always good to have on hand, provided they're all-natural and low in sodium.

Focus on seasonal and local. The nutritional density of recently, locally picked food is superior to food that was picked before it was ripe, shipped across the world, kept in cold storage and then delivered to your grocery store where who knows how long it may have sat in the storage bin. (More in Chapter NINE).

Continue to check nutrition labels even for products you regularly buy; companies often change recipes, ingredients or contents while keeping the packaging the same.

Keep copies of pre-printed lists handy. Write a template. List your three favourite vegetables, fruits, lean proteins, nuts and seeds and whole grains. Print duplicate copies. Then add and subtract to the list each week as needs arise.

 Phase III: SHOPPING

Supermarkets can be dangerous neighborhoods. Here are some tips to protect you on your journey:

Shop with a list. Remember: nothing in the grocery store is there by mistake. Even the height of the shelf on which an item is placed is designed to entice you to buy it. Be wary of any item you want to buy that isn't on your list.

Don't shop when you're hungry. Big mistake! Items you know you don't normally eat or don't need will suddenly appear in your cart/home/stomach.

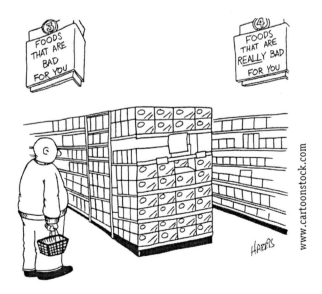

CHANGE4GOOD – ACTION STEPS

- Start implementing Principle 6 – Read: Those Tricky Food Labels.
- Clean and Unclutter Kitchen: cupboard, pantry, fridge and freezer (and your mind).
- Write a weekly meal plan or plans and grocery list(s); shop.
- Identify and complete your fifth short-term (weekly) goal. For example: Buy user- (and environmentally) friendly containers for portioning out and storing food. Buy a basket in which to keep mail and bills.
- Complete your Change4Good Nutrition GPS©.
- Update Change4Good Journal daily©.
- Update Change4Good Goal Sheet weekly©.

TOOLS

- Change4Good Goal Sheet©
- Change4Good Journal©
- Change4Good Grocery List©

REMEMBER THIS

- Buy foods appropriate for your Garden of Eden.

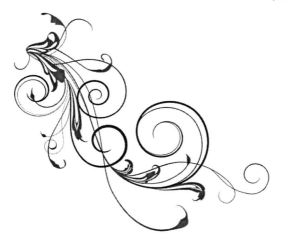

READY, SET, MODERATE

This chapter is about right-sized eating, drinking – and thinking.

Principle 7 Manage: Food and Beverage Portions

Listen to your body. Easier said than done – but if you do, it will reward you with health and well-being. Feel satiated but not full to the point of discomfort. The best way to determine the size of your portions; is your hand.

"Believe you can and you're half way there."
~Theodore Roosevelt, 26th President of the United States of America

PORTION MANAGEMENT

I have a friend, a former dancer, who wanted to maintain a healthy weight and did not, like so many dancers, want to live a life dominated by an eating disorder. Her solution; "I only ate three-quarters of what was on my plate."

Personally, I'd find not finishing what was on my plate torture but it worked for her. For those of you like me, who can't leave even a grain of rice (especially if it's nutty brown and lightly drizzled with flaxseed oil), **there's a better method: take less.**

Learn to know how it feels to fulfill your body's requirements. But beware: it takes at least 20 minutes after eating to accurately gauge how really full you are. Of course most of us eat beyond this point. As a result, we skip the stage of feeling comfortably satisfied and jump right into "stuffed". This chapter will help you learn how to stay at comfortable and avoid that "oh no" feeling the next morning.

Just for the record – we now know what *standard food serving sizes* **are for the various types of macronutrients:**

- **Protein 30 grams**
- **Starchy/complex carbohydrates 15 grams**
- **Fats 5 grams**

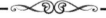

Take less and learn to know how it feels to fulfill your body's requirements. It takes at least 20 minutes after eating to accurately gauge how really full you are.

Portions, on the other hand, are how much you now choose to have at your meals and snacks. For example my portion of protein at lunch, which may be the size of the palm of my hand, would be the equivalent of about 3 servings of protein – or 90 grams as one serving of protein is 30 grams. My portion of rice may be the size of my fist – about ½ cup, which would be about 1.5 servings of carbohydrate.

As with all the other tools of the program, portion control need not be complicated nor time consuming. It does, however, have to be consistent. Various methods and tools can help.

1. **The method I have found to be most successful is the simplest: your hands.** They're a marvelous guide to insuring that you get enough – but not too much – food.

2. **Another simple rule: keep a half-cup measuring cup and a tablespoon measure on your kitchen counter as well.**

3. Finally, **learn to listen to your body** (tricky since our minds are not always our friends).

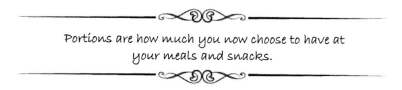

Portions are how much you now choose to have at your meals and snacks.

To eat well you don't need to weigh food down to the last milligram. As a result, the Change4Good system is discrete and eminently transportable. It works in a tent camping out; it works at the latest Michelin multi-star restaurant in France.

1. Hands On

   Always compare what you have on your plate to the size of either your palm or your fist. When using the palm of your hand as a guide, it is the length, thickness and width of your palm, the part in which you'd catch a ball.

    1 portion of leafy greens or non-starchy vegetables should be what you can fit in two cupped hands (remember non-starchy vegetables can be added freely to any meal or snack – you can essentially eat as many non-starchy vegetables as you like).

    1 portion of fruit and starchy / complex carbohydrates from whole grains or starchy vegetables should be the size of a clenched fist.

    1 portion of meat or other protein should be the size of the palm of one hand.

    1 portion of healthy fats should be about the size of your thumb but this will vary, depending on the source, from 1 teaspoon to 2 tablespoons.

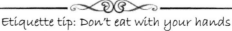

Etiquette tip: Don't eat with your hands
– but do measure with them.

More on Fats:

- 1 teaspoon = 5 grams or 5ml (examples include olive oil, flaxseed oil, butter, ghee).
- 2 teaspoons = 10 grams or 10ml (nut butters, tahini, reduced fat mayonnaise).
- 1 tablespoon = 15 grams or 15ml (seeds, cream cheese, regular oil/vinegar salad dressing).
- 2 tablespoons = 30 grams or 30 ml (half/half cream, sour cream, reduced fat cream cheese, reduced fat oil/vinegar dressing).
- Nuts are different sizes but a rule of thumb (no pun) would be about 5-10 nuts or 1-2 tablespoons. A few more for pignoli, and a few less for big nuts like Brazil nuts. But 5-10 nuts are a safe amount.
- Remember to also trim all visible fat off food before cooking.

When dinner arrives, discretely look at your fist and see whether you've been served the right amount.

If you're eating out, unless you are dining in five star restaurants (which are known for their small portions), chances are you have more protein and carbohydrate than you need and of course, far fewer vegetables than you need.

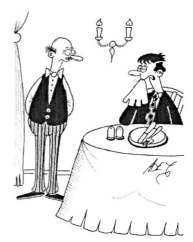

"How did I find my steak? well I lifted up a roast potato and there it was."

www.cartoonstock.com

2. *Counter Couture*

Keep a half-cup measuring cup and one tablespoon measure on your counter. Why? Because otherwise, it's so easy to overeat cereals, grains, yogurt, oils, salad dressings and soft cheeses. If the half-cup and tablespoon measures sit there permanently, you'll be more inclined to use them.

How easily we can convince ourselves that the bowl of cereal we just ate was half a cup when in fact it was more like a full cup or more. These "little" extras, unfortunately, add up to the one pound or ten we seem prone to gain. I'm so in the habit of using my half cup measuring cup (cooked rice, oatmeal, yogurt, even ice cream) it's practically my third arm.

3. *Listen to Your Body*

Remember Principle 1: Eat intentionally? **You cannot be conscious of how much you are eating and how it makes you feel while multitasking.** As we said in the previous chapter, eating and driving/talking/texting/watching television are out.

Mindful eating works better and for two reasons:

- First, so you can be aware of how full you are.
- Secondly, so you can actually enjoy the experience which will affect the satisfaction – and therefore the level of physiological satiety – or fullness – you feel. And how should you feel? To the point where you feel satisfied – could definitely eat a little more – but know that it's not required.

Personally, if I'm concentrating too hard on anything but the meal before me, then when I'm done I'm usually stunned; "Good grief! There's nothing left."

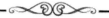

Eating is an art. The more you settle into it, the more it will favour you with satisfaction.

The antidote is to listen to relaxing music while you eat. Eat slowly. Even if you flip through a magazine or re-think your day, make sure you take time out to relish the art of eating delicious food. Gratitude also helps: not everyone has the luxury of struggling to eat quality foods in appropriate quantities.

Listening to your body also means learning to differentiate between physical hunger and emotional appetite. We've discussed this aspect of eating in Chapter THREE, but simply put, remember: hunger is the true physical need for food. Appetite is the emotional need for food. If your need is emotional, no portion control strategies are going to help.

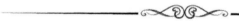

Listening to your body also means learning to differentiate between physical hunger and emotional appetite.

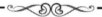

Another point worth repeating: make sure it's food you need and not water, as previously discussed (Chapter FIVE). Most people find out it's really water they need. If, on the other hand, you're hungry and you're eating the prescribed 4-6 meals/snacks a day, chances are they're missing some important macro-nutrient (Protein? Carbohydrate? Fat?) or they're not nutritionally dense. Zero-calorie gelatine or low-"point" desserts won't do much to satiate real hunger. **Respect your body. Don't try to get away with giving it junk – even of the low-cal sort.**

The Age of the '–chinos

These days, it seems as if everyone walks around holding a cup, as if it were a part of one's anatomy. Bad news: unless you're drinking water or herbal teas, you're probably slurping calories.

Most adults have given up sugary sodas (not that the diet stuff is anything you'd want to pour into your body). And most of us (with of course exceptions) leave alcohol for dinner or social gatherings.

But what about all those coffee-plus beverages out there – the lattes, frappachinos, mochachinos and other adult "milkshakes." Even Chai tea with low fat milk has about 200 calories.

These drinks have calories and sugar and, what's worse is they stimulate your appetite for more of the same. The solution; relegate coffee-shakes to the 10 percent part of the 90/10 rule (See Chapter EIGHT, Principle 8). And don't kid yourself: milk is mostly sugar; these drinks are not particularly nutrient-dense. As for calcium, there are better, less addictive sources.

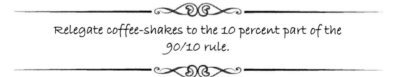

Relegate coffee-shakes to the 10 percent part of the 90/10 rule.

Other Portion Management Strategies

Below – additional visual cues that may help you manage your portions.

1 Meat/Poultry serving (3 oz.)	1 Portion = size of a deck of cards or Blackberry®
1 Fish serving (5 oz.)	1 Portion = size of a check book
1 Fruit serving (½ cup)	1 Portion = size of a tennis ball
1 Starchy Vegetable serving (½ cup)	1 Portion = size of a tennis ball
1 Grain/Cereal serving (½ cup)	1 Portion = size of a tennis ball
1 Dairy serving (8 oz.)	1 Portion = the size of a container of individual yogurt
1 Fat serving (1-2 tsp.)	1 Portion = ranging between the size of a dice and a ping pong ball

 Size Up (Down) Your Dishes

Since the 1970s, dinner plates have increased in size by about 25 percent (from about 10 inches in diameter to 12 inches). People trained or accustomed to "cleaning up" their plates are eating more without even realizing it. Brian Wansink, PhD., of Cornell University says that if you eat off a plate about 2-inches smaller, you will serve yourself 22% fewer calories per meal, which translates into a 2-pound weight loss in one month. Not only will you eat less but because the plate appears fuller, you will feel like you are eating more – a truly win-win situation.[18]

One sensible solution might be to use your salad plates for higher-calorie meats or pastas, and your dinner plate for salads and vegetables. Or, buy dinner plates that are 10-inches in diameter. His findings apply to serving utensils as well – use smaller serving spoons – and glassware.

According to Wansink, people – even professional bartenders – pour more of a beverage when using short, wide glasses than they do when using tall, skinny ones. The reasons? We tend to focus on the height of beverages when pouring, not the width or cubic volume. Pouring just 2 extra ounces of orange juice every morning could result in a gain of three pounds a year.

The easiest solution is to start using skinny glasses for calorie-laden drinks and wider ones for water. You could lose one pound in six months just by cutting out one sugar-sweetened drink serving per day.[19]

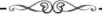

Solutions: use your salad plates for higher-calorie meats or pastas, your dinner plate for salads and vegetables, and use skinny glasses for calorie-laden drinks and wider ones for water.

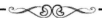

And if you're into gadgets, here are some that aid in portion control that are fun:

- Ceramic Design for Health Portion Plate®
www.jeffreyharris.net/products.aspx
- Plastica Bento Box®
www.plasticashop.com
- Measure Up Bowl®
www.shopmeasureupbowl.com
- Digital Spoon Scale®
www.spoonsisters.com
- Wine-Trax glass®
www.wine-trax.com
- Flavour Magic Portion Control Sheets®
www.portioncontrol.net

Portion Distortion: Here are five additional situations that Wansink identifies that can greatly distort your perception of how much you eat:

1. **You're sitting at the dinner table, surrounded by serving platters.** Not surprisingly, you're more likely to pick even after you're done. And picking is dangerous. I had a relative who used to "sliver" a cake to death.

   A better option is to plate your main dish (protein, veggies, and starches) and, if it's your house, immediately store the leftovers. You're less likely to automatically go for seconds if the food is not easily accessible. On the flip side – keep salads and vegetables on the table during dinner as most people do not eat enough vegetable servings per day.

   If you're out, move the excess food to a separate plate and ask to have it wrapped "to – go". That way, you don't feel like you're being cheated out of what is rightly yours.

If you're eating at someone else's house and you can't quickly store away the food, do so mentally. Engage in a conversation with someone. Mentally, prepare to eat one small plateful and then look forward to herbal tea or fruit.

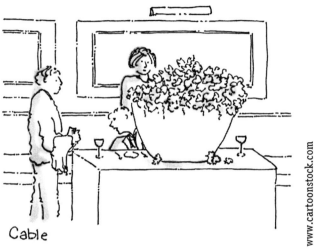

Cable

www.cartoonstock.com

"We've decided to split the Caesar salad."

2. **Supersized-packages are almost as dangerous as super-sized plates.** Brian Wansink found that people ate twice as many candies from big bags as from smaller ones, regardless of the candy. Big packages fool you into thinking you've hardly made a dent in them. Better to break them down into smaller containers or single-serving portions before you begin eating, and put the rest away.

3. **Visibility of food is also an issue.** Wansink also found that secretaries told to eat as much candy as they wanted out of a clear bowl averaged two more candies per day than those given the candies in an opaque bowl. Similar results were seen with proximity of candy – the closer it was the great the quantity that was eaten. The moral of this story? Should you keep unhealthier snacks around, keep them out of sight.

4. **Calorie, fat and quality of nutrients also affect how much we eat.** People tend to eat more when they know a food is considered low calorie, low fat, healthy or organic. Don't fool yourself. Healthy food has calories too.[20]

5. **Variety is also un-helpful.** Domenica Rubino, M.D., director of the Washington Center for Weight Management and Research in Virginia, has found that the more variety of food we are exposed to, the more we are likely to eat as we taste a little of each to see which we prefer. By having only one choice, you will eat less and enjoy that item more.[21] Fewer choices let you savour the flavour of one particular food.

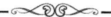

The more you cultivate the habit of eating the right amount, and that may include tweaking your social life or environment, the more successful you will be.

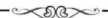

What about alcohol?

You need to pay as much attention to alcohol portions as you do to everything else. **Alcohol contains about 7 calories per gram or 73 calories per ounce.** Below is a listing of what are considered standard sizes for a single drink. Although they are different sizes they contain approximately the same amount of alcohol but calories vary from between 100–150 calories per serving.

> 12 fl. oz. of regular beer
> 8-9 fl. oz. of malt liquor
> 5 fl. oz. of table wine
> 3-4 oz. of fortified wine (such as sherry or port)
> 2-3 oz. of cordial, liqueur, or aperitif
> 1.5 oz. of brandy (a single shot)
> 1.5 fl. oz. shot of 80-proof spirits/hard liquor (whiskey, vodka, gin, tequila, rum)

Women should limit their total alcohol intake to **no more than 7-9 drinks per week** and **men no more than 8-13**, ideally not having more than 3 drinks in one sitting more than once a week.

Although these "standard" drink amounts are helpful for following health guidelines, as with food, they may not reflect customary serving sizes. For example, a single mixed drink made with hard liquor can contain 1 to 3 or more standard drinks, depending on the type of spirits and the recipe. **Therefore, proceed with caution and your liver (and waistline) will thank you.**

"Discipline it the bridge between goals and accomplishment."
~Jim Rohn

FOOD AND MEAL PREPARATION STRATEGIES

In Chapter SIX we discussed what to buy. Now we'll talk about what to do with it. The shopping experience doesn't end when you simply unpack your groceries at home. Now's the time to flip on the news or radio, or turn on your favourite sound track and work: wash, cut, chop, put in re-sealable zipper storage bags and cook foods that can be prepared ahead of time and stored in the fridge or freezer.

A drag; it merely requires establishing new habits. Start allowing time to prep vegetables and fruit and other fresh produce the day you buy it. Set aside time each week to do some bulk food preparation – while your favourite show is on the radio or television or you're listening to a great book on tape. **Try and make food preparation a positive experience.** You'll get to savour these moments and to grow attached to that large bowl of crudité waiting for you in the fridge every night.

Keep less perishable snack foods like nuts and seeds or rice cakes already doled out into portion-controlled containers. I never make rice for one or two or even four. I make it for six or eight and then stow away appropriate portions in Ziploc® bags and freeze it. Ditto for soups; cool them and then ladle into leak-proof containers and freeze. Then all you need to do is remember to take it out in the morning; and if you forget, there's always the microwave.

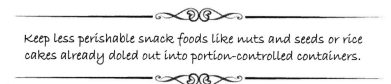

Keep less perishable snack foods like nuts and seeds or rice cakes already doled out into portion-controlled containers.

For the super busy (or lazy), buy pre-cut veggies and salads in bags. They aren't as tasty but on a day when you have a board meeting or a paper due, they'll taste just fine.

Change4Good Basic Kitchen Gear List©:

Now for the fun part: food preparation kitchen gadgets. These will not only make food preparation easier, but more efficient and fun. But before you head out to the store for your new "toys," consider the types of foods you regularly cook and only get what you need. If you never eat cheese, no need to by a cheese grater.

◯ **Appliances**:

- **Blender**: great for smoothies. But first – see below:

    A word about smoothies: Make them at home and they're as pretty and as satisfying as any drink you buy with a–"chino" at the store. And note not only the money and calories you save but the nutrients you gain.

    - Quick smoothie snack: protein powder and almond/rice milk.
    - Quick smoothie meal: protein powder, almond/rice milk, Greek (higher protein) yogurt, frozen and/or fresh fruit, and water – maybe a bit of flax seed oil for those healthy Omega-3s.

    I drink meal-size smoothies as either breakfast or lunch. Protein powder you say? That's not real food. Well, yes, it isn't, but life being what it is, one does occasionally have to do something for the sake of convenience.

    As mentioned in Chapter FOUR, protein powder, without additives, is a quick and healthy source of low-fat protein. Remember to buy the kind without added sweetener or other gunk. Refer to the Change4Good Grocery List© at **www.change4good.ca** for specific brands that are both healthy and tasty.

- **Crockpot or slow cooker:** great for soups and stews – even oatmeal so it is ready for your early breakfast.

- **Food processor:** big and/or small.

- **Indoor grill.**

- **Rice cooker/steamer:** preferably with ceramic or stainless steel lining.

- **T-Fal Actifry**®: now you can enjoy your sweet potato fries guilt-free.

- **Wok:** oil free magic: add water or a bit of balsamic vinegar or Bragg's All Purpose Seasoning®.

Containers:

- Casserole dishes
- Freezer bags
- Storage containers (Oven/freezer-friendly)

Utensils:

- Baking sheets
- Cookware set
- Knives
- Mixing bowls
- Stainless steel tools
- Water Filter Jug
- **Vegetable peeler** (buy the best you can - saves hours and finger tips)
- Cutting board
- Graters
- Measuring cups and spoons
- Spatulas
- Strainer
- Wooden spoons

Putting those Gadgets to Work:

Before you get started, here is a list of flavourings from the Change4Good Grocery List© to add some healthy flavour to your cooking: To download the complete and regularly updated list with some recommended brands go to **www.change4good.ca.**

Change4Good Seasoning List©

Seasonings | dressings, hoisin sauce, lemon juice, mustard, pasta sauce, soy sauce, tobasco sauce, tomato paste, vanilla extract, vegetable broth, vinegar – balsamic, rice, red wine etc.
spices/herbs: bay leaves, black pepper, dried basil, mint, oregano, ground cinnamon, cumin, onion powder, paprika, salsa, salt alternative, sea salt, etc.

Keep a batch of grilled vegetables on hand. Use your indoor or outdoor grill. If you have them, believe me, you'll use them. Eat as either a snack, or add to salads, omelettes or as a side to your dinner. Grilled shitake mushrooms (drizzled with balsamic vinegar or a dash of Bragg's All Purpose Seasoning©) improve EVERYTHING.

Cooked foods store beautifully too. Cook for armies even if you're only one. As previously mentioned, regarding rice, soup, stews: cook and cool. Then pour one or half-cup portions into re-sealable zipper storage bags or plastic containers and freeze.

Stock up on Protein:

- **Start with eggs.** Hard boil and store in the fridge. They'll keep for up to five days. But what about cholesterol you ask? If you don't have a cholesterol issue, you can safely eat one or even two a day. Remember, eggs contain lecithin. It's good for you and it helps break down the cholesterol in the egg.

Avoid frying. Instead, poach, boil or scramble. In addition to adding calories, oil at high temperatures oxidizes cholesterol.

- **Chicken next**. If you eat chicken, cook a half dozen breasts at once, freeze or store in the fridge – then get creative. Do a chicken salad one night, a stir-fry another, and finally, take a chicken breast in a pita sandwich with vegetables to work.

- **Beans:** Soak overnight then cook up a pot for the next week. A great idea is to simmer with a square of kombu, a type of seaweed you can buy at your local gourmet or health food market that adds flavour and a tad of healthy ocean salt. Then store in the fridge or freeze in bags. Throw in soups or microwave and add to salad or rice. In a pinch, use canned beans; they are just as nutritious and more convenient.

- **Nuts/seeds:** I always keep a supply in re-sealable zipper storage bags. I measure out an ounce or two and then grab a bag when I'm on the run. Packed this way, nuts are healthy, ready to go and because they're pre-portioned, you won't eat too much of this otherwise good thing.

A note on freezing: label the package with the item, the serving/portion size (e.g. 1 cup of soup, two grilled chicken breasts) and the date.

Prepare dinner (fully or partially) before you leave for work so it's waiting there with open arms when you walk in all frazzled or even elated after a long day.

With or without gadgets, you're all set to implement Principle 7 - Manage: Food and Beverage Portions. You're conscious now of what an appropriate portion looks like. No more wondering why that one bowl of ice cream (three cup-fuls really) is making you gain weight. Or why a cappuccino really doesn't provide sufficient protein for a meal. Again, look at your hand before you eat, and make sure your plate contains: a palm-size of protein; no more than a cupped palm or half cup size of a cooked grain; two palm-fuls of vegetables; a thumb-print of oil or fat.

Then: Wait twenty minutes after you eat. Are you really hungry? You won't be if you've eaten not too much or too little of the right foods. Chew slowly. Sip water and give thanks for the beautiful meal your body is preparing to savour and eat.

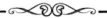

Look at your hand before you eat, and make sure your plate contains: a palm-size of protein; no more than a cupped palm or half cup size of a cooked grain; two palm-fuls of vegetables; a thumb-print of oil or fat.

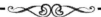

CHANGE4GOOD – ACTION STEPS

- Start implementing Principle 7 – Manage: Food and Beverage Portions.
- Do the opposite of what your mother said – use your hands (for measuring only). See if you have an appropriate amount of protein, carbohydrate, fruit, fat and vegetables on your plate.
- Implement at least three new food preparation strategies.
- Identify and complete your sixth short-term (weekly) goal. For example, "I'll prepare a pot of soup and freeze in 1-2 cup portions. I'll buy a top of the line vegetable peeler."
- Complete your Change4Good Nutrition GPS©.
- Update Change4Good Journal© daily.
- Update Change4Good Goal Sheet© weekly.

TOOLS

- Change4Good Goal Sheet©
- Change4Good Journal©
- Change4Good Basic Kitchen Gear List©
- Change 4Good Grocery List©

REMEMBER THIS

- Fast food comes in two forms – good and bad. Avoid the latter by always keeping on hand a ready supply of the former.

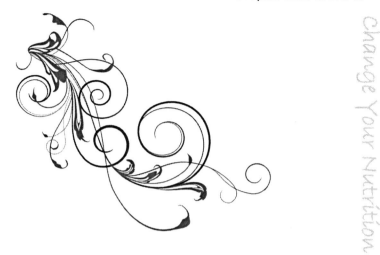

Chapter EIGHT

OUT AND ABOUT: DOING IT ON THE ROAD

Whether in Paris, Rome or an island in the Caribbean, eating sanely makes your holiday more – not less – pleasurable.

Principle 8 Practice: Moderation; Follow the 90/10 Rule

Change4Good isn't anti-pleasure. It's pro-pleasure, on the assumption that when you limit the "fun" stuff, you enjoy it more and it harms you less. Eating healthily 90% of the time makes you appreciate the "fun" foods more and "want" and "need" them less intensely.

> "If one oversteps the bounds of moderation,
> the greatest pleasures cease to please."
> ~Epictetus, Greek Sage and Stoic Philosopher

Although statistics vary in terms of actual percentages, it is well know that North Americans are eating out more and more. No wonder, given our hectic lives. We eat in hotels and in restaurants, at food courts, business meetings, buffets and family gatherings. In most of these circumstances, we have little, if any, control over what food is served and how it's prepared. For most people, a change of circumstance is like a "get out of jail" key. Oh, good, we think; time to go off my diet. That's where Change4Good comes to the rescue. You're not on a diet. **Your eating is a way of life. Eat healthy 90% of the time, and then go enjoy your 10% "off".**

The irony, as I mentioned, is that once you begin to regularly incorporate healthy eating into your life, your desire for treats won't extend much beyond that 10%. A slice of cheesecake and a glass of wine on a Saturday night will probably sate it.

90/10 is another way of saying: avoid the all-or-nothing attitude. You cannot have it all - the bread, the wine and the dessert. But you can decide to have your individual non-negotiable foods – what you are not prepared to give up. Once you decide upon those, work around that decision.

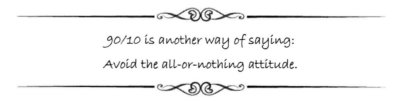

90/10 is another way of saying:

Avoid the all-or-nothing attitude.

Some of my clients say they cannot give up their glass of wine at dinner. Others cannot resist dessert. Still others cannot end a meal without a latte (more than 100 calories – and that's with skim milk). That's fine. Just work it into your plan.

On a recent night out, after scanning the menu, I decided I could live without the French onion soup, and the bruschetta with avocado and feta, but I'd have to have the crème brulee for dessert – with a tea. And I did (yum). And because I ate healthily the rest of the day and didn't skimp on protein or veggies at dinner – I had grilled tilapia, and stir fried vegetables—I wasn't famished by the time I got to the crème brulee. Had I skimped on dinner in order to "save room" for dessert, that first bite of crème brulee may have set up a craving and who knows if one serving would've been able to satisfy it?

This chapter will provide you with "practice" at eating out, showing you specific menu selections and teaching you effective strategies to choose among them. Sometimes, the choices aren't good (ever tried eating healthily at a baseball game?) **All you can do in some circumstances is what you always only have to do: the best you can.**

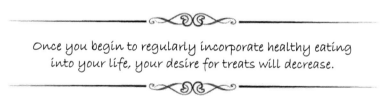

Once you begin to regularly incorporate healthy eating into your life, your desire for treats will decrease.

Eating out doesn't only mean wining and dining in restaurants. It also means eating outside of your kitchen and comfort zone on days that bring you out of your routine. Most recently Tuesdays were my very busy days: I taught 8:30-11:30am. After an hour break, I taught again from 12:30-6:30pm. No time for food? Right? Wrong. Years of experience have taught me that the last thing I want to do at night is walk into my kitchen half crazed with hunger and fatigue. My antidote; I plan ahead.

Monday night I ask myself, "How many meals or snacks am I going to need tomorrow?" Then I check the fridge. Once I've figured out my strategy, I whip out my journal (by now, it should be your custom– see Principle 2), and write down a plan. I may not stick to it perfectly but having it there works wonders in implanting it in my brain. That night or the next morning, I pack what I need.

Lauren's Menu for Tough Tuesdays:

Breakfast:	Protein-rich oatmeal pancake (1/4 cup uncooked oats; ½ cup egg whites; 1 tbsp. ground flax seeds). Use a non-stick pan; fry and pack. Some days I'll spread a little organic jam on it, but I've actually grown to like it plain.
Lunch:	Small can of tuna that I mix with salsa; one sweet potato, and cut up vegetables, including some avocado – all packed in a plastic container.
Snacks:	Two fruits, usually a banana and an apple (I pick fruits that are easy to eat). Plenty of water. Maybe a healthy snack bar (see Change4Good Grocery List©) or some Babybel® cheese and 10–12 almonds.

Now when I walk into my kitchen, I'm calm enough to enjoy a cup of tea. At the very least, I'm calm enough to relax while I prepare dinner (veggie burger with stir fried vegetables – frozen if I'm lazy— and maybe fruit and a yogurt for a late night snack). The food tastes great – when you're hungry, healthy food always does – and I'm blessed with a feeling of satisfaction that extends beyond the food. Now, on to other things because life is not only about our meals; it's about what we do in between them.

Prête à Porter (Ready to Go)

Some people might despair at all the work and advance planning involved. Not me. If I didn't take my (snazzy purple insulated) lunch sack to the college where I teach, Tuesdays would mean greasy pizza or stir-fry in the student cafeteria. Ugh. Why pay for high-calorie food that I don't even like?

Now, to get you started. Here's the equipment (edible and non-edible) you'll need on hand to make eating on the run easy:

First, a cooler bag or find something functional that works for you. In addition to your cooler bag you will also need:

- Ice packs to keep your food cool.
- Napkins.
- Reusable containers in which to seal your food.
- Reusable water container – I toss this into my briefcase.
- Thermos for soups.
- Utensils.
- Ziploc® bags.

If you can't pack a cooler for the entire day, at the very least toss a few nutritious snacks and foods into Ziplocs® that you can keep in your purse or briefcase: raw nuts, dried fruit, and good snack-bars (see the Change4Good Grocery List© at **www.change4good.ca**). Armed with these accoutrements, you're health and well-being are safe anywhere.

Remember tips we discussed in earlier chapters: cook extra food at dinner so you have leftovers to eat the next day. It takes as much effort to grill four chicken breasts as it does eight; to boil twelve eggs instead of four; to make a large pot of rice versus a small one. And of course, remember that ever-ready bowl of washed and cut vegetables, into which you're dipping, I trust, every day.

Staples I select from for my cooler

- Almonds (10 - 12 per serving)
- Almond milk
- Babybel cheese
- Berries (fresh or frozen)
- Cottage cheese
- Grains (cooked rice, quinoa)

- Hardboiled eggs
- Hummus
- Kefir

- Pre-cut vegetables

- Ricotta cheese
- Snack bar such as Vega®/Lara®/Elevate Me®

- Yam/sweet potato

- Almond butter
- Apples
- Bananas
- Chickpeas with salad dressing
- Fruit Salad
- Grilled fish (salmon, trout and tilapia to name a few)
- Herbal tea bags
- Kashi Go Lean Cereal®
- Plain Greek yogurt (highest protein and least carbohydrates)
- Protein powder (see Change4Good Grocery List© for recommended brands)
- Ryvita® crackers
- Water-packed tuna mixed with salsa/cottage cheese or salad dressing

You now have enough variety to create several good-for-you meals and snacks to pack into your cooler bag and to sustain you on the road. Even at a hotel or business event, how nice it is to have all this body-friendly food, leaving room for you to enjoy a nice dinner out, if that's what your business – or pleasure – requires.

RESTAURANTS AND FOOD COURTS (Uh-oh)

Fortunately restaurants are more accommodating than ever before. First, I'll show you what I do when dining in a place I adore, and second, I'll give you 10 strategies to take with you for the rest of your eating-out life.

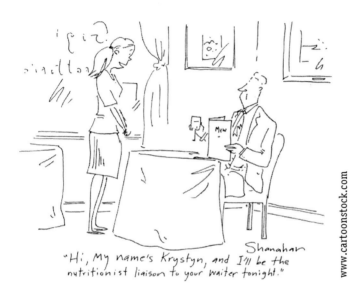

"Hi, My name's Krystyn, and I'll be the nutritionist liaison to your waiter tonight."

www.cartoonstock.com

Shanahan

Remember: The best choice may simply be
the best of what's available.

Practice: Moderation; Follow the 90/10 Rule

Dinner at Your Favourite Restaurant

Here I am at one of *my* favourite restaurants, which I frequent
in summer because of its lovely patio.

⟳ Appetizer Ruminations:

I could eat the entire list: sweet potato fries; feta
bruschetta and spinach and roasted garlic goat cheese dip
with Nacho chips and warmed pita. Instead, I order the
edamame. I'm saving my calories for dessert
(cheesecake).

⟳ Pondering L'entrée:

I'll choose either the grilled salmon with Portobello
mushrooms and bell peppers on a bed of baby spinach
(dressing on the side, please) or the fish of the day or a
veggie burger (hold the bun) – each with a side salad.

Here's what I'm *not* going to eat: the Caesar salad and/or
the New York strip steak (the smallest is 10oz) or the
beef burger (smallest is 9oz) – still holding out for
dessert.

⟳ Operation Dessert:

I'm going for the cheesecake (with tea). Some other time,
I'll have the baked apple-raspberry pie or flourless
chocolate cake. Because I've eaten prudently during the
rest of the meal, I could really choose any dessert I
please. Cheesecake (my favourite) is usually among the
more caloric choices. Sometimes, I'll coax my dining
partner into sharing it with me.

◯ To Drink:

Some of you would trade cheesecake for a scotch on the rocks or a gin and tonic? Fine; just steer clear of drinks with mixers (double the calories). Another caveat: some people lose their inhibitions while drinking. If wine makes you overeat, avoid or sip it slowly throughout the meal. I also sip water with lemon.

Restaurant Tool Kit

- Do not arrive hungry – the best of intentions will be hard to follow if you arrive famished. However counterintuitive, munch something small and nutritious an hour or so prior to dining – a small apple and a slice of cheese, a half cup of yogurt – just to take the edge off.

- Plan accordingly – have lighter meals and snacks throughout the rest of the day, cutting back on complex/starchy carbohydrates and fats – but don't go on any kind of severe diet. Avoid at all costs *the big build up.*

- Do your homework – most restaurants post menus on line, and most fast food chains (McDonald's®, Subway®, Starbucks®) post nutritional charts. Read these in advance and plan. In dining out as in life, spontaneity is sometimes dangerous.

- Call ahead for special meals or requests - most restaurants will accommodate them especially if made in advance. Also, making arrangements by phone saves you time and in some cases, the discomfort of having to explain your nutritional needs in front of business associates or friends.

Practice: Moderation; Follow the 90/10 Rule

- Avoid the bread basket - unless it's going to be part of your 10% treat; ask your server not to bring it.

- Monitor the extras - when ordering salads, ask for scant dressing or dressing on the side. Skip the croutons. Remember, ketchup and mayonnaises have calories, too. Depending on the quality of the restaurant, you may want to ask for sauce on the side. In a three-star French restaurant, the sauce may be worth lapping up but in many cases, the food tastes better without it.

- Be specific when you order - state clearly that you'd like your fish plain broiled. Look for items that are baked, dry, broiled, steamed, poached or grilled; served in broth or with marinara, white wine or a tomato based sauce. Unless you're really determined to splurge, avoid the white stuff (Alfredo, Béchamel sauce).

- Avoid over-ordering - consider what you would have if you were home. Would you really fix yourself an appetizer, main course and a dessert? Then why do it when you are dining out (unless one of these is part of your 10% allowance)?

- Don't forget your hands - they'll help you assess portion size. Alternatively, you can share an entrée; select both your appetizer and main course from the appetizer section or ask for half of a whole portion to be packed to take home before it is served. And dessert, of course, is always a share-able pleasure with half the guilt.

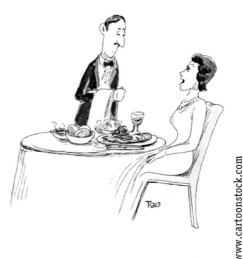

"I'll pay double for half as much."

www.cartoonstock.com

Change Your Nutrition

- Eat slowly - remember that important fact: it takes your brain 20 minutes to inform your stomach that you are full. When in doubt, stop. Also, pace yourself. You don't want to finish eating before everyone else. People who do find it almost impossible not to nibble. Chew properly (it's better for digestion); sip water; pause; rest; set down your knife and fork every once in a while. All these techniques are centering. They help you remember you have a mind and a heart that need feeding at this meal, not just a stomach.

Change4Good Menu Cheat Sheet©

Menu

Beverages – water, club soda, limit to one alcoholic beverage, maximum two

Appetizers – broth-based soups, edamame, green salad dressing on the side, lean protein (grilled calamari, satay stick)

Salads – dressing on the side, or use vinegar/olive oil/lemon juice, avoid croutons, bacon, processed cheese

Sandwiches – choose wholegrain bread, use mustard instead of butter/mayonnaise/cheese, limit dressings, sauces and spreads, fill up on vegetables, choose lean protein (lean beef, grilled chicken, turkey)

Entrees – broiled, dry, baked, grilled low-fat protein (seafood, chicken, fish, lean beef), ask for entrees to be prepared without butter and sauces – or have sauces served on the side

Side Dishes – plain/steamed vegetables without butter/sauces, avoid sour cream

Dessert – fresh fruit, low-fat latte/cappuccino

Pay special attention to descriptions on menus:

- Low-fat/calorie indicators: au jus, baked, broiled, dry-sauteed, flame-cooked, grilled, marinara, poached, roasted, smoked, steamed
- High-fat/calorie indicators: alfredo, au gratin, batter dipped, béarnaise, béchamel, beurre blanc, bisque, breaded, carbonara, casserole, creamy, crispy, en croute, escalloped, flaky, fried, gravy, hollandaise, parmigiana, puffed, tempura

NAVIGATING A BUFFET

The never-ending buffet is some people's dream and my nightmare. **Steel yourself by studying the following:**

- Look before you leap - see what's there. Prioritize, just like you would at home if studying a menu on line before going out to a restaurant.

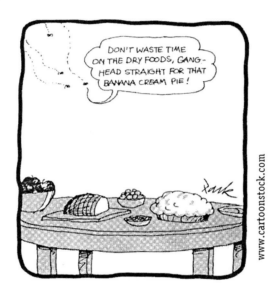

- Don't stand and eat - some people think that food that you eat while standing "doesn't count." It does in terms of calories although not always in terms of satisfaction.

- Always have water to drink at your table.

- Green salad ingredients are almost always available but limit yourself to only two sources of fat in your salad – for example avocado and dressing or nuts and dressing.

- For your main course, choose one lean protein and one complex carbohydrate and plenty of vegetables. Although it's fun to sample and taste, you tend to eat more with greater variety on your plate. As in life, I'm afraid, you have to limit yourself: one carbohydrate and one protein, but feel free to go wild with the vegetables (provided they're un-sauced).

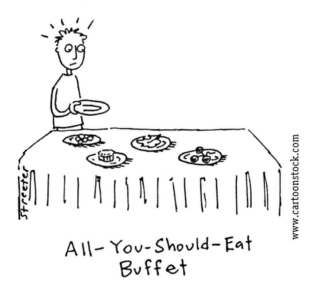

www.cartoonstock.com

All-You-Should-Eat
Buffet

- Fool yourself - use a salad plate as your dinner plate.

- The good news about buffets: there's almost always fresh fruit for dessert.

- Last but not least, your neighbour's plate is none of your business. Don't be influenced by what or how much s/he is eating. Keep the focus on yourself and your goals.

EATING OUT AT THE HOMES OF FRIENDS AND/OR FAMILY; ENTERTAINING, HOLIDAY MEALS AND SPECIAL OCCASIONS

All these events are tricky because they test your people skills too. Are you prepared to say "no thank you" to the host; or to insult your Aunt Ruth by turning down a piece of her famous pie? By comparison, restaurants are easy. The chef doesn't care if you re-design an order – or you don't know if he does – but a relative; or a friend? This is where you will need to practice "tough love".

Here are additional tips:

- First and foremost, focus on the people and conversation, not the food.

- Occupy your hands with a glass of water or a spritzer, and occupy your mind with good conversation and friends, to avoid the temptation of finger-foods and hors d'oeuvres, which are generally loaded with calories and fat.

- Ask what will be served so you can plan appropriately if you're dining with family or friends, and if you feel comfortable – your sister-in-law is used to your eating habits by now – certain situations are more conducive to soliciting the host's help in advance than others. There are situations in which I've even nibbled on a salad and sipped Perrier, but did my major eating at home.

- Offer to make something – and then make a dish you know you can eat as well.

Practice: Moderation; Follow the 90/10 Rule

- As at buffets and in restaurants, prioritize. You can't have all the hors d'oeuvres, side dishes, desserts and wines, and still stay fit, so pick and choose. How nice you'll feel the next morning, remembering the great conversations you had instead of bemoaning the bathtub of calories you consumed.

- If a special holiday food is offered only this time of year, enjoy it. Remember a treat is different from a binge. Avoid extremes. Revel in moderation.

- If you're the host, be the clean-up squad too. Get rid of unhealthy leftovers. Give them to guests or throw them out. Freeze or put away healthy leftovers so that you don't mindlessly pick.

- Keep up your exercise routine (even though it's the holidays or a special event).

- Keep journaling (ditto the above).

More on the 90/10 Split

In terms of food (and beverages), **the 90/10 split suggests that you allow yourself a treat meal/food/drink each week (hold the guilt).**

Before you rush off to obtain it, let's look a little more carefully at the meaning of 10%. Say you are eating 5 meals/snacks each day; that will be 35 meals/snacks per week. Ten-percent of 35 are 3.5 meals/snacks. In other words, approximately 3 times per week you are not just permitted – you're required – to have a treat (on the theory that the flip side of deprivation is over-indulgence).

Not surprisingly, the 90/10 rule is the most popular Change4Good Principle©. Sometimes, it's helpful to schedule or plan your treats. Spontaneity is nice but not always when it comes to treats.

Trick or treat?

Some clients prefer to use their entire 10% on alcohol. They have 2-3 drinks a week spread out in any form they choose. It may be one or two mixed drinks, three glasses of wine; maybe three cans of beer (see Chapter SEVEN for portion control); either all in the course of one long evening event or at various times throughout the week.

Other clients go strictly for dessert. I fall into this category. Almost every weekend I eat some kind of dessert – crème brulee substituted occasionally for my beloved cheesecake. I also love pizza, but frankly, I almost prefer the healthy kind: multi grain, thin crust; vegetables galore, and cheese only as a light dusting. Pizza for dinner means: two to three small slices and a salad.

Of course once you're at a healthy weight, an extra treat occasionally won't throw off your system. More indulgence than that, though, will do dangerous things to your mind.

Some people want me to parse the 10% down into calories. I refrain. Obviously a hefty slice of a chocolate layer cake is going to out "weigh" two moderate glasses of white wine in terms of calories. My best advice: use common sense.

An extra treat occasionally won't throw off your system. More indulgence than that, though, will do dangerous things to your mind.

Punishment Fitting the Crime

Some unhealthy "dieter" types get around the 90/10 rule by substituting a treat or two for an entrée or even an entire meal. Sorry – the rules don't allow it. If you don't eat any protein one day, you lose one of your three treats. Skip your 2.5 litre of water ration? Off comes another treat.

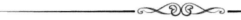

Sometimes, it's helpful to schedule or plan your treats.
Spontaneity is nice but not always when it comes to treats.

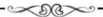

CHANGE4GOOD – ACTION STEPS

- Start implementing Principle 8 – Practice: Moderation; Follow the 90/10 rule.
- Incorporate three treats this week and record (in your journal) how it went.
- Pack a cooler for the next appropriate occasion (business trip, long day at the office).
- Identify and complete your seventh short-term (weekly) goal. For example, "I will research the online menu of my favourite restaurant; buy a funky cooler bag; make a selection of non-perishable pre-portioned and packaged snacks".
- Update Change4Good Journal© daily.
- Update Change4Good Goal Sheet© weekly.

TOOLS

- Change4Good Goal Sheet©
- Change4Good Journal©
- Change4Good Menu Cheat Sheet©

REMEMBER THIS

- The 10 Change4Good Principles©: Don't leave home without them.

Chapter NINE

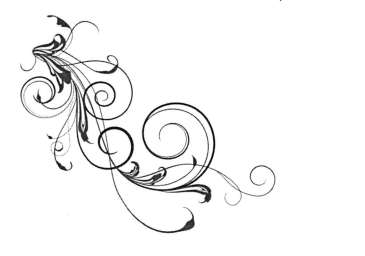

LUXURY PROBLEMS: TAKING NUTRITION AND HEALTH TO THE NEXT LEVEL

Here's everything you need to know about detoxification and cleansing, supplements, organic food consumption, vegetarian diets and pH balance.

Principle 9 Drink: 1 - 2 Litres of Water Every Day

Start with warm water and lemon first thing in the morning (the water stimulates the colon; lemon cleanses the liver) and keep at it all day. One litre equals slightly more than 4 cups. Remember: losing weight and then maintaining a healthy weight also depends on adequate hydration.

"When you reach the top, keep climbing."

~English Proverb

Out in the "real world" there's a lot of buzz about this next level, which includes concepts like detoxification and cleansing, eating an all-plant diet, and taking supplements – to name a few. You're curious. Voodoo? Or gospel? You want to know. Unfortunately, there's a lot of misinformation about these concepts as well. In this chapter, I'll give you reliable information about all of these advanced callings, using as our guide, as always, the key term: moderation.

Before you start, assess your progress so far. Go through the Change4Good Progress Checklist© below, answering honestly. When gauging your success, subject each to the 90/10 rule: have you been following it 90% of the time for at least the past 3 months?

Assessment: Change4Good Progress Checklist©

1. Do you eat 5-13 servings of vegetables each day? (Remember: ½ cup cooked or raw is a serving).   YES   NO

2. Does your breakfast include at least protein and complex carbohydrates (e.g. egg whites and whole grain toast, almonds and oatmeal)?   YES   NO

3. Do you eat 4-6 small nutrient dense meals/snacks per day?   YES   NO

4. Do you prepare most of your meals and snacks yourself?   YES   NO

5. Does each meal include sources of lean protein, a healthy fat and natural carbohydrate?   YES   NO

6. Do you check food labels (surprised that that "all natural" oatmeal packet is loaded with sugar)?   YES   NO

7. Do you keep yourself properly hydrated (1-2 litres/day) and drink more water when you work out?   YES   NO

8. Do you avoid processed, refined foods and alcohol 90% of the time?   YES   NO

9. Do you order primarily nutritious food at a restaurant or when eating out?   YES   NO

10. Do you monitor your food portions?   YES   NO

If you answered, "no" to any of the questions – go back and implement the particular principle(s) in which you're falling short. Try to understand why you are not implementing them.

If you answered, "yes" to seven questions or more – congratulations. You're living the principles. You're ready to kick it up to the next level.

Remember, moving on to this next section is not an all-or-nothing proposition. You can decide to go vegetarian one day of the week only at first (if at all). You can implement just a few of the cleansing/detox principles – your call. Just (again) be moderate.

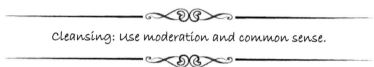

Cleansing: Use moderation and common sense.

ARE YOU READY FOR A CLEANSE/DETOX?

First, let's distinguish between the two. (Mainstream articles often confuse the two.)

A detox helps remove toxins from the body and is usually organ-specific; for example, a liver detox cleans out the liver; a kidney detox cleans out the kidney. Depending on the organ cleansed, different supplements and products are used. An organ-specific detox can be intense and have serious side effects; it is best undertaken with a trained and certified health practitioner. Also, it isn't quick. **Thorough detoxing could take weeks or even months rather than days.**

A cleanse, on the other hand, is simpler, focusing mainly on clearing and cleaning the digestive tract; its goal is to rid the body of parasites and fungi (like Candida) and the bowels of toxic, compacted fecal matter. Some toxins are released, but not all.

Many methods used for one can also be used for the other:

- Eating a diet of organic fruits and vegetables cleanses the colon by way of increasing (as in a colon cleanse, the increased propels the elimination of toxins via fecal matter).
- Consuming only organic fruits and vegetables introduces nutrients into the body, which accelerates its natural detoxification process.

Both a detox and cleanse allow the body to catch its breath. I use a gentle cleanse with many of my clients. About 99% of them say that when they go back to eating normally after the cleanse, much of the food that they ordinarily ate no longer tastes as good. They want to eat more healthily. And that's after only one week. It shows how quickly your taste buds can change to provide you with what your body wants.

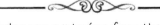

A detox helps remove toxins from the body and is usually organ-specific. A cleanse focuses on clearing and cleaning the digestive tract.

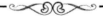

Opinions of traditional health practitioners on both of these processes vary. Some see a benefit; others, not. Personally, I think the colon cleanse is healthy and beneficial for most people, and the few supplements it requires can be part of a year round regimen. (See cleansing process below.) After all, how bad could it be to free your body from processed foods for a week?

In this chapter, we'll mostly focus on cleansing the digestive system. It's a good idea to do a digestive/colon cleanse before doing a specific organ detox, anyway, because if your colon cannot efficiently get rid of the waste – which contains many of the toxins being released – detoxification can actually do more harm than good.

Just for the record: we're discussing physiological cleansing methods, but the term is useful in terms of our mental and emotional states as well. As we saw in Chapters ONE and THREE, it may be as important to cleanse your mind – of negative thought patterns – and your environment – of harm or stress – as it is to cleanse your body. Remember that, now, back to the physical realm.

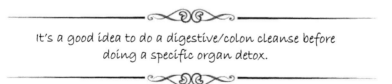

It's a good idea to do a digestive/colon cleanse before doing a specific organ detox.

Toxins, Toxins Everywhere

What are Toxins?

They're any substance that undermine or stress optimal functioning. **We're all exposed to toxins that affect our health on a daily basis.** They usually accumulate in our fat cells, our weaker tissues, glands and organs; our lymphatic tissue and along the walls of the intestines, especially the colon. Their build-up results in numerous illnesses, health complications and weight gain. We cleanse (or detox) to stimulate the body to release – get rid of – stored toxic wastes.

Every day, our bodies detoxify naturally. A person's ability to detoxify is partly based on genetics. For example, if you have a weak liver, the organ primarily responsible for detoxification, your body will have a harder time detoxifying than the body of someone with a healthier liver.

Under normal circumstances, our body handles toxins in several ways:
- It can neutralize them (via antioxidants).
- Transform them, like the liver does, into harmless substances.
- Eliminate them, like the kidneys do.
- We also clear toxins through sweating from exercise or heat.

Anything that supports elimination can be said to help us detoxify.

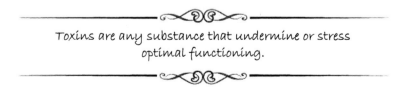

Toxins are any substance that undermine or stress optimal functioning.

Detoxification helps the body's own, natural cleaning process.

Here's how:

1. Through fasting or a modified diet, it allows the organs to rest.
2. It stimulates the liver to drive out toxins.
3. It promotes elimination through the intestines, kidneys and skin.
4. It improves the circulation and cleansing of the blood.
5. It refuels the body with healthy nutrients.

The major parts of our body involved in physical detoxification are, not surprisingly, those involved in the cleansing process naturally:

- **Digestive tract**
- **Liver**
- **Kidneys**
- **Skin**

An additional system involved that we haven't mentioned is the lymphatic system. It's a secondary circulation system (blood being the primary one). The lymphatic system does not have a pump (like the heart) to aid its flow. It relies upon muscles to stimulate its circulation.

The lymphatic system serves several purposes.

- First, it **maintains the fluid balance in our body** by collecting excess fluid from tissues and returning it into the bloodstream. Without it, massive edema (swelling due to accumulation of fluid) would occur causing tissue destruction or death.

- Second, it **produces lymphocytes** (a type of white blood cell), which form part of our immune system.
- Third, it **filters out foreign substances** such as bacteria and toxins.
- And finally, it **absorbs fats from the intestine and transports them to the bloodstream.**

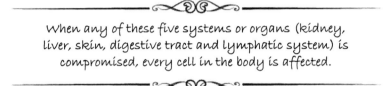

When any of these five systems or organs (kidney, liver, skin, digestive tract and lymphatic system) is compromised, every cell in the body is affected.

How to Cleanse

The best time to follow either a cleansing (or detoxification) program is in the spring and fall – due to less extreme weather. Also consider what's going on in your life. Don't do it during a particularly stressful time in your life. Remember, cleansing doesn't have to be an all-or-nothing process. Select your first step and then move forward at a pace that suits you.

If you've never done one before, I'd do the one recommended in this book (gentle cleanse). Try it for 7 days or 5 or 3 – any amount is better than none. Also, don't do a cleanse more than twice a year. Generally, a complete regimen should last from between a week to ten days maximum.

There are dozens of different cleansing programs: some last days, others weeks. Some require a change in diet; others, fasting.

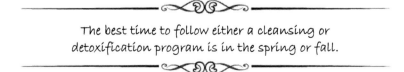

The best time to follow either a cleansing or detoxification program is in the spring or fall.

Fasting doesn't actually cleanse the colon; it merely gives the digestive system – small intestine and related organs (liver, gallbladder and pancreas) – a rest so that the body can focus on healing and repairing as opposed to its every-day hard work of digesting and absorbing food.

- A water fast (most extreme and not recommended) eliminates all food.
- A juice fast (less extreme), eliminates solids. In a juice fast, the ingestion of high quality nutrients (both fruits and vegetables that are liquefied) stimulates the cells to release the poorer quality nutrients it may contain – like spring cleaning (you throw out your old clothes and make room for new ones).

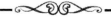

Fasting doesn't actually cleanse the colon; it merely gives the digestive system a rest so that the body can focus on healing and repairing.

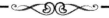

The least extreme or gentle cleanse involves a less restrictive diet of water, juice, vegetables and fruits. Some regimens also use herbs, supplements and other elements.

A cleanse specifically for the colon helps rid the colon of all waste matter. It can be done via colonic water irrigation – similar to an enema – or through supplementation of fibre and acidophilus (healthy bacteria naturally found in our colon which help in human digestion). In cleaning out the colon, a colon cleanse may also clear toxins out of other cells in the body as well. A juice fast, on the other hand, doesn't clean out the colon due to a lack of fibre.

Indicators of Toxicity

Almost everyone experiences some of these symptoms of toxicity listed below. And just because you do, doesn't mean you're "toxic," merely that it's a possibility. However, it's always good to rule out physiological causes first. If one or more of these symptoms persist for at least six months and to the extent that it disrupts your normal routine, your body may be telling you it's sick.

- Frequent fatigue
- Chronic constipation
- Excess weight
- Powerful food cravings
- Frequent colds and flu
- No sense of purpose
- Wide mood swings
- Insomnia or sleeping too many hours

- Compromised digestion
- Skin eruptions
- Poor stress management
- Depression
- Recurring headaches
- Pain in joints
- Self-defeating belief systems

Before you embark on a cleanse or a detox, consult with a qualified health practitioner – especially if you are on any medication or have severe health problems. Do not undertake a cleanse or detox if you are pregnant or breast-feeding.

On the next page are **a list of items to remove from your diet,** and **a list of items to include every day.** If you are following the 10 Change4Good Principles©, you are probably already consuming (and avoiding) the right stuff.

Items to REMOVE from your diet *(if you already haven't)*:

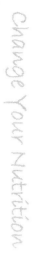

- **Highly processed foods** (table sugar, white bread, luncheon meats and frozen dinners).
- **Poor quality oils** (partially hydrogenated or those with trans-fats).
- **Fruits and vegetables that have been irradiated, sprayed, waxed or dyed.**
- **Deep-fried or barbecued meat.**
- **Food additives and preservatives.**
- **Excessive caffeine and stimulants.**
- **Artificial sweeteners.**
- **Refined salt.**
- **Soda** (including seltzer and sparkling water).
- **Commercial milk and milk products** (inorganic).
- **Commercial meat** with hormones, antibiotics (as opposed to organic and grass fed).
- **Empty calorie, non-nutritious food.**
- **Genetically Modified Food** (not required to say on the package but usually it tells you if it isn't).

Items to INCLUDE in your diet:

- A wide variety of **natural, nutrient-dense foods.**
- **Pure water and herbal teas.**
- **Healthy fats** (Omega-3, 6 and 9).
- **Fish and seafood from deep-water** areas.
- **Natural sea salt, organic herbs and spices.**
- **Foods that support balanced blood sugar** (i.e. unprocessed and with low GI or GL).

Eat organic products as much as possible (more on organic food later in this chapter); at the very least, eat local and seasonal produce. Also, avoid foods that you know you have trouble digesting (i.e., some people may have a hard time with legumes or cauliflower, for example).

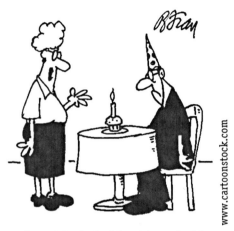

"IT'S WHEAT-FREE, DAIRY-FREE, FAT-FREE, NUT-FREE, SUGAR-FREE AND SALT-FREE...ENJOY!"

Change4Good One-Week Cleanse©:

On the next page is a gentle cleanse that I have used with hundreds of clients. Again, it's simple but not necessarily easy. Almost everyone who does this cleanse reports feeling healthier, lighter and more energetic after a week.

In any cleanse, you'll need to drink lots of water to flush out all the toxins and accommodate the increased fibre intake. Luckily, this week's Change4Good Principle is to drink 1–2 litres of water a day. Remember, the one-week cleanse plan is only suggested. Feel free to adapt it to your needs and level of commitment. Note, too, that although supplements might aid the cleansing process, they aren't essential.

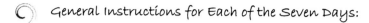

General Instructions for Each of the Seven Days:

- **Begin each day with a glass of warm water and a teaspoon of lemon juice/slice of lemon.**
- **Eat only natural, whole and unprocessed foods** during this time, preferably organic.
- **Drink at least 4-8 glasses of water per day;** herbal teas can also be included.
- **Do not overeat.**
- Try to **wait 3 hours between meals.**
- **Get plenty of rest.**
- **Make your own salad dressing** to use on vegetables if necessary.

Here is an easy salad dressing recipe:

In a bowl, stir together all the ingredients, making sure they are well mixed:

1 tsp. flaxseed or olive oil

3 tsp. lemon juice or apple cider vinegar

Pinch of Celtic/sea salt or Herbamare

Serve chilled. This dressing is best used within a few days of making.

Cleanse Plan

Day 1	Fruit, raw or cooked vegetables, whole grains (brown rice, quinoa, millet), sweet potatoes and yams
Day 2	Raw fruit and vegetables
Day 3	Raw vegetables*
Day 4	Raw vegetables*
Day 5	Raw fruit and vegetables
Day 6	Fruit, raw or cooked vegetables, whole grains (brown rice, quinoa, millet), sweet potatoes and yams
Day 7	Fruit, raw or cooked vegetables, whole grains (brown rice, quinoa, millet), sweet potatoes, yams and protein (preferably fish) or protein powder

Drink: 1–2 Litres of Water Every Day

* NOTE: If you find the vegetable-only days too challenging, add some fruit. Also, if you need to, lightly steam your vegetables or make a vegetable soup to add a bit of variety.

Beets, radishes, artichokes, cabbage, broccoli, spirulina, chlorella, and seaweed are all excellent detoxifying foods.

Sample Change4Good Cleanse Menu Plan©:

	Upon Waking	Breakfast	Lunch	Dinner	Snacks
Monday	warm water & lemon	mixed berries	steamed vegetables & brown rice	grilled vegetables with a yam	fruits & vegetables
Tuesday	warm water & lemon	fruit salad	spinach salad with mango & berries	kale salad with avocado	fruits & vegetables
Wednesday	warm water & lemon	vegetable juice (carrot, celery, parsley, spinach)	chopped vegetable salad	steamed spinach with mushroom & asparagus	fruits & vegetables
Thursday	warm water & lemon	vegetable juice (tomato, kale, cucumber, cilantro, lemon wedge)	steamed vegetables (steamed broccoli with olive oil & lemon juice)	chopped vegetable salad	fruits & vegetables
Friday	warm water & lemon	fruit salad	grilled vegetable salad	broccoli salad with avocado	fruits & vegetables
Saturday	warm water & lemon	banana & berries	steamed vegetables with quinoa	grilled vegetables with wild rice	fruits & vegetables
Sunday	warm water & lemon	kiwi & pineapple	brown rice salad (rice with vegetables)	green salad with grilled fish	fruits & vegetables

Cleanse Reactions:

The body may initially react to a cleanse. In general, the worse your diet, the more you'll feel the effects of the cleanse. Take heart: the body's reaction is a good sign, a clear indication that your body is responding. The reaction usually lasts for a couple of days, depending on the kind of cleanse and the initial level of toxicity. It may also be a reaction to the withdrawal from stimulants like caffeine and sugar regularly consumed in the diet.

Symptoms may include:

- fever
- muscle and joint aches
- constipation
- gas and bloating
- diarrhea

- headaches
- fatigue
- skin eruptions
- bad breath
- mood swings

Persist and eventually you will feel more energized and healthier.

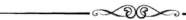

The worse your diet, the more you'll feel the effects of the cleanse. Take heart: the body's reaction is a good sign, a clear indication that your body is responding.

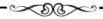

Another way to assist the cleansing process is to stimulate the circulatory and lymphatic systems of the body. A few reliable methods:

1. *Showers*: End your shower by having a few minutes of comfortably hot water followed with a rinse of icy cold water for several minutes.

2. *Epsom Salt Baths*: Epsom salts help eliminate toxins by increasing blood supply to the skin and drawing toxins from the body. Add 1-4 cups to tub. Soak no longer than 30 minutes.

3. *Dry Skin Brushing*: Use a long handled natural bristle skin brush. Do this before you shower or bathe for about 5 minutes starting at your feet and working upwards with small circular movements. Finish with your stomach and brush in a clockwise direction to stimulate the digestive tract. Do not brush too hard.

4. *Massage*: Certain types of massage techniques help stimulate your body to release stored toxins. **"Swedish Massage,"** for example, tends to stimulate massaged cells to release stored toxins. **"Lymphatic Massage"** helps circulate lymphatic fluid throughout the body. If you get a massage, drink plenty of water for at least the next couple of hours; the extra water will help the kidneys quickly rid the body (through urination) of the new toxins in the blood and lymphatic fluid.

5. *Mini-Rebounder*: Rebounding helps both the immune and the lymphatic systems operate more efficiently. At the top of each jump (on a mini-trampoline), you achieve a weightless state; then land with twice the force of gravity. The change in gravitational forces experienced during rebounding allows for greater blood flow, which in turn increases the amount of waste products flushed from the cells. Rebounding can increase lymph flow by up to 15%.

It also conditions and strengthens the heart which allows the resting heart to beat less frequently. Researchers at the University of Kentucky, in conjunction with NASA, concluded that "the magnitude of the biomechanical stimuli is greater with jumping on a trampoline than with running" and that it is 68% more efficient than jogging.[22]

Implementing these activities in your daily routine has been shown to cleanse and strengthen cells, stimulate the lymphatic system and improve circulation. These are also a great way to start your day. You won't just look better; you'll feel better too.

Supplements, too, can enhance the cleansing process

The choice of supplements will depend on the type of cleanse you are doing and your goals. Again, these are optional and should be approved by a qualified health care practitioner (i.e., one who is licensed by a reputable program. Don't hesitate to check credentials on the web).

Some recommended cleansing supplements are included on the Change4Good Supplements for Health List© on page 273. But first a caveat, always use the previously suggested Change4Good Cleanse Menu Plan© as opposed to anything provided in these kits. See further information on supplements in general below.

Once you have completed your one-week cleanse, continue on your regular eating plan, following the usual 10 Change4Good Principles©. Continue certain aspects of the cleanse – drinking warm water and lemon every morning – long term.

Drink: 1-2 Litres of Water Every Day

To Supplement – Or Not

Ideally we want to get our nutrients from foods. They provide our bodies with the ideal mix of vitamins, minerals, enzymes, antioxidants and energy, and in the appropriate proportions. When you isolate specific nutrients as in multiple vitamin supplements, you lose that so-called "synergy". You are only getting part of the whole thing.

In addition, researchers have hardly identified all the nutrients that exist in food – although they've identified many of them. For this reason, among others, **almost no vitamin or pill can ever replace real food.** Taking pills only gives us the nutrients scientists have been able to identify, isolate, analyze and replicate – only a fraction of what's in food.

Having said all that, I'll put in a pitch for supplements as well, but only after you've filled yourself with as much nutritionally-dense food as your caloric intake allows.

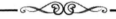

Ideally we want to get our nutrients from foods. They provide our bodies with the ideal mix of vitamins, minerals, enzymes, antioxidants and energy, and in the appropriate proportions.

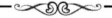

As their name indicates, "supplements" are only intended to *supplement* what we can't obtain from food. Perhaps we don't eat enough fruits, vegetables or fish high in Omega-3. Or perhaps the quality of the food we eat isn't as nutrient-dense as formerly, the result of soil depletion, poor agricultural practices and pollution. **Many aspects of agribusiness now focus on appearance rather than nutritional content of a food. As a result, even eating a healthy diet may leave us nutritionally deficient.**

And while it's true that no supplement can compensate for an overall poor quality diet and lifestyle, some supplements may fill the gap in even the most healthy food plans.

Principle 4 instructs you to include healthy fats in your diet each day. Yet, Omega-3s are difficult to obtain from our daily food. Most people will need to supplement with Omega-3s. It is estimated that the majority of North American adults are Omega-3 deficient.

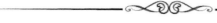

As their name indicates, "supplements" are only intended to supplement what we can't obtain from food.

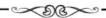

Regarding fruits and vegetables, you face similar problems. Few of us eat the necessary amount of fruits and vegetables, which are ideally, 5-13 servings a day. And in order for those to be optimally beneficial, the items would need to be organic and locally grown, and your body would need to be able to digest and absorb them properly. No wonder we're supplement-happy.

The Change4Good Supplements for Health List© provided on page 273 is by no means all-inclusive, but it does provide you with a list of general categories of basic supplements that most people may need at some point but certainly not all of them all of the time.

Remember: we're all different. Your needs should be assessed based on your blood work, symptoms, history and goals, and should be determined by a qualified practitioner.

Remember: just because a product is natural doesn't necessarily mean it's safe. Also, beware of mixing items. Contraindications can occur amongst different supplements and between supplements and medications.

Here are some general rules to keep in mind while taking supplements:

1. *Divide the dose throughout the day to maximize utilization.* One exception is Vitamin D.

2. *Take with food for maximum absorption and utilization.* An exception is iron, which you should take on an empty stomach, and only if a blood test confirms that you have low levels. Another exception are amino acid supplements; these, too, are best taken on an empty stomach.

3. *Take B vitamins earlier in the day* (they increase energy) and as part of a B complex, since B's work best in concert.

4. *Make sure mineral supplements are chelated,* which means they are bound to small protein building blocks/amino acid, which will enhance absorption across the intestinal wall and into the bloodstream.

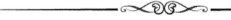

Just because a product is natural doesn't necessarily mean it's safe. Contraindications can occur amongst different supplements and between supplements and medications.

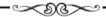

Research Roulette: Are Vitamins Actually Helpful?

Research in science and particularly in nutrition, of course, changes constantly. We come across new findings and disregard old ones. With that caveat, bear in mind that there is valid, independent, published, peer reviewed research showing that taking certain isolated vitamins and minerals may not be so helpful and in some cases, harmful.

- One study of 15,000 physicians, found no difference in heart disease in men taking Vitamins E and C compared to those taking a placebo.[23]

- Another study failed to show that Vitamin E and selenium supplements change the risk of developing prostate cancer in older men.[24]

- In addition, some research has shown that mega-doses of vitamins may actually be harmful. An analysis of randomized-controlled trials (the gold standard in research design) found that people who take antioxidant supplements, especially Vitamin A, beta carotene, and Vitamin E, had higher mortality rates, while Vitamin C and selenium supplements seemed to provide no benefit or harm.[25]

The results on studies with multivitamins are no better.

- The Women's Health Initiative Study (February 2009) published in the Archives of Internal Medicine found that after eight years of taking a multivitamin, 161,000 older women showed no difference in their rates of heart disease and cancer.

  The study provided convincing evidence that multivitamin use has little or no influence on the risk of common cancers, CVD, or total mortality in postmenopausal women.[26]

- And most recently (March 2010), a study published in The American Journal of Clinical Nutrition showed that multivitamin use was associated with a statistically significant increased risk of breast cancer. [27]

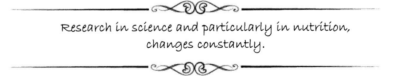

Research in science and particularly in nutrition, changes constantly.

Overall, most studies have shown no significant association between most isolated vitamin supplements and improved health. Three exceptions are:

- Folic acid supplementation in pregnant women to prevent pregnancy complications.
- Calcium in the prevention of bone loss. (More discussion on calcium and bone loss further ahead in this chapter).
- Vitamin D in the absorption of calcium and phosphorous to prevent bone loss.

Note: There are new supplements on the market that, unlike vitamins, do not contain isolated nutrients but instead, contain whole foods, for example, in one case, a combination of 17 different whole fruits, vegetables and grains that have been juiced, dehydrated and encapsulated.

The goal of these is to help bridge the gap between the amount of fruits and vegetables our bodies need and what we actually consume and absorb. I'd recommend these instead of a multivitamin. Also of interest are so called "greens" supplements. Although made of natural ingredients, they are however, still man-made formulas and lack the synergy of real food.

True confession: From time to time, I do take and recommend isolated nutrients, but only to temporarily support specific symptoms or nutritional imbalances. Currently the only individual vitamins I take regularly are a D3 Vitamin and an Omega-3 Fish Oil Supplement. In addition to this, I also take Juice Plus® which is one of the few "whole food" supplements on the market.

Not immune to "health fads" myself (!), I have recently added
to my daily protein shake Maca, a root vegetable food that
grows in Peru. It is an herb that acts like an antioxidant and
supposedly: increases the body's ability to adapt to stress;
helps regulate the endocrine system; improves energy and
stamina and enhances memory, mental clarity, fertility and the
regulation of hormonal imbalances. Do we know that it in fact
does all these things? No, but it's one of the latest
"superfoods" in the nutritional literature – and allow me my
indulgences; at least it's not cheesecake (which as you know, I
occasionally indulge in too).

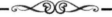

*Overall, most studies have shown no significant
association between most vitamin supplements
and improved health.*

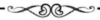

Supplements for Health

One final concern: the vitamin and supplement industry isn't
currently standardized and dietary supplements are regulated
under different rules to conventional medications.

**According to the FDA and Federal Trade Commission's website,
dietary supplements do not need approval from the FDA before
they are marketed. There are currently no provisions in the
law for the FDA to "approve" dietary supplements for safety or
effectiveness before they reach the consumer.**

Manufacturers are however expected to ensure their products are safe but based on numerous product recalls over the years, we know this is not always the case.

So, unless you know which supplements are proven and of quality, you may be wasting your money and putting yourself at risk. Fortunately, in Canada this scenario is currently changing and much stricter regulations are being put in place to protect consumers.

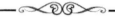

The vitamin and supplement industry isn't currently standardized and dietary supplements are regulated under different rules to conventional medications.

In the meantime, below are a few general guidelines. To insure that any supplements you do take comply with at least certain safety regulations and are those of maximum quality, **look for at least one of the following numbers on their labels:**

- D.I.N. (Drug Identification Number)
- N.P.N. (Natural Product Number)
- G.P. (General Product)
- U.S.P. (United States Pharmacopoeia)

Keep in mind though that these standards indicate quality, purity and tablet disintegration – not how bioavailable and effective they are.

In addition, you can refer to **MedlinePlus®** which is the National Institute of Health's website, produced by the National Library of Medicine. Here you have **access to information about the effectiveness, usual dosage, and drug interactions of many dietary supplements and herbal remedies.** However these recommendations are not brand specific.

Now, always taking the above into careful consideration, on the next page is a list of supplement categories, I recommend to many of my clients. Again, I suggest you consult your health practitioner before you start any supplementation regimen to determine what is safe and necessary for your particular situation. For a regularly updated list of specific brands please go to **www.change4good.ca.**

The Change4Good Supplements for Health List©

Supplement	Benefit
*Whole Food Nutrition	Essential for overall health, general nutritional balance, source of antioxidants, vitamins and minerals.
*Greens	Essential for overall health, general nutritional balance, source of antioxidants.
*Chlorophyll	Detoxifies and cleanses blood, activates immune system, antioxidant benefits.
Spirulina	Antioxidant benefits, activates immune system.
Maca	Adaptogen (reduces stress impact on body), improves energy, hormonal balance, metabolism, fuels endocrine system.
Essential Fats Omega-3 With 1000mg EPA and DHA	Assists with every function in the body from heart health, to hormone regulation, to brain function etc.
Flaxseed Oil	Assists with every function in body from digestion, cardiovascular health, cancer fighting etc.
Digestive Enzymes	Assists with digestion of food and increases absorption of nutrients.
*Probiotics	Improves intestinal health and increases healthy bacteria in the colon, aids digestion.
*Fibre	Cleanses colon, decreases appetite, stabilizers blood sugar.
B Vitamins Take before 2pm	Stress and mood management, energy production, nervous system maintenance.
Vitamin D	Bone formation, absorption of calcium and phosphorous, enhances immunity, mental wellness.
Calcium/Magnesium	Bone formation/maintenance, transmission of nerve impulses, muscular contraction, blood clotting etc.
*Total Body and Colon Cleansing Kits	Assists in total body organ and colon cleansing.
*Liver Cleansing	Help to support the functioning and cleansing of the liver.

*These supplements will specifically assist when doing a cleanse. With the advice of a health care provider, select which is most appropriate for your goals and/or condition.

Bone Up: The Case for Calcium

Increasingly, people are living longer. Their bones, unfortunately, don't always keep up with other parts of their bodies. This is especially true in Western cultures. For that reason, in recent years, many doctors have prescribed calcium supplements to their clients, especially female clients. Of course the best source of calcium is, always, food. Milk is the most popular, but it has a high level of phosphorous, which makes the calcium in it harder to obtain. Below is a list of calcium-rich foods other than milk (it includes both dairy and non-dairy items).

It is suggested that adults get between 1000-1200 mg/day; for post-menopausal women, the dosage is up to 1500mg, although there is controversy about that as well. Some practitioners advocate less calcium through supplementation and a diet richer in plant protein. Also, it is important to note that the amount in milligrams of calcium in foods other than milk varies; different sources give different numbers. I've chosen the ones most commonly cited.

Calcium-Rich Foods from Sources Other Than Milk

Dairy foods (all low fat)

- ¾ cup of yogurt – 300-400mg of calcium
- ½ cup ricotta cheese - 337mg
- ¾ cup kefir – 225mg
- 1 ounce of mozzarella – 183mg
- ½ cup of cottage cheese– 69mg

Milk Alternatives

- 1 cup soy milk (fortified) – 300mg
- 1 cup rice milk (fortified) – 240mg
- 1 cup almond milk (fortified) – 200mg

Protein foods

- 3 ounces canned sardines (with bones) - 340mg
- 1 cup regular tofu (uncooked) - 260mg
- 3 ounces canned salmon (with bones) - 200mg
- 1 cup tempeh (cooked) - 154mg
- 3 ounces trout – 75mg

Nuts and Seeds

- ¼ cup almonds - 100mg
- 1 tablespoon sesame seeds - 90mg
- 1 tablespoon flaxseeds - 90mg
- ¼ cup brazil nuts – 65mg
- 1 tablespoon almond butter – 43mg

Legumes

- 1 cup soybeans (cooked) - 175mg
- 1 cup kidney beans (cooked) – 69mg
- 1 cup chickpeas (cooked) – 76mg
- 1 cup black beans (cooked) – 46mg
- 1 cup lentils (cooked) 37mg

Fruits

- 5 dried figs - 135mg
- 1 orange - 50mg

Vegetables

- 1 cup collard greens (cooked) - 220mg
- 1 cup bok choy (cooked) – 158mg
- 1 cup broccoli (cooked) - 94mg
- 1 cup kale (cooked) - 90mg
- 1 cup butternut (cooked) - 90mg
- 1 cup sweet potato (cooked) – 64mg
- 1 cup broccoli (raw) - 42mg

Drink: 1-2 Litres of Water Every Day

If you do take calcium supplements, make sure they are in a chelated form such as calcium citrate, calcium lactate, and calcium gluconate – these are all better absorbed by the body than other forms such as calcium carbonate. Your calcium supplement should also contain magnesium and Vitamin D to aid in absorption.

Also check the amount of elemental calcium to evaluate the actual amount of useable (although not necessarily absorbable) calcium in the supplement. **To retain maximum supplement absorption take only about 500mg or less at one time.** Also check with a pharmacist that there can be no adverse interactions with any other supplements or medications you may be taking.

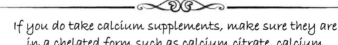

If you do take calcium supplements, make sure they are in a chelated form such as calcium citrate, calcium lactate, and calcium gluconate.

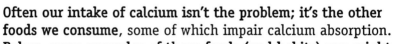

Often our intake of calcium isn't the problem; it's the other foods we consume, some of which impair calcium absorption. **Below, some examples of those foods (and habits) you might wish to avoid:**

- *Sodium:* Salt increases the amount of calcium excreted in the urine. If you're eating foods high in salt, eat more calcium or better yet, cut down on salt.

- *Excess protein:* As protein is burned for energy, it produces sulfate. Sulfate increases the amount of calcium excreted in the urine, which decreases the amount of calcium in the body. Excess protein creates excess sulfate.

- Oxalate: Found in some foods and beverages, most notably spinach, chard, berries, chocolate, and tea, oxalate binds with calcium and increases the loss of calcium through fecal excretion. For example, even though sweet potatoes contain calcium, not all of it is absorbed because of the oxalic acid (oxalate) they contain.

- Phytic Acid: Another plant chemical that inhibits calcium absorption, phytic acid is found in the hulls of grains, seeds, and nuts. It is the main way that plants store the mineral phosphorus. Cooking reduces phytic acid, as does soaking the foods in an acidic medium such as lemon juice, or fermenting or sprouting foods.

- Phosphorous: Also known as phosphoric acid and phosphate, phosphorous, which is in cola and many processed foods, can interfere with calcium absorption. Cow's milk has a fair amount of phosphorous which can interfere with the absorption of the calcium in milk. When eating a calcium-rich meal, best to avoid even diet drinks and seltzer.

- Insoluble fibre: This type of fibre, such as the kind in wheat bran, reduces calcium absorption.

- Alcohol intake: Drinking excessive amounts of alcohol can interfere with the calcium balance by inhibiting the enzymes that convert inactive Vitamin D to active Vitamin D.

- Caffeine: excessive intake of caffeine (300-400mg) can increase urinary excretion as well as fecal excretion. (One cup or 8 fl. ounces of brewed coffee contains about 137mg of caffeine).

Smoking, stress, and lack of exercise: These lifestyle factors also contribute to the body not being able to absorb calcium as efficiently.

The most significant nutrient needed for the proper absorption of calcium is Vitamin D; it comes from two sources:

- First, it is made in the skin through direct exposure to sunlight.
- Second, it comes from the diet.

The body's ability to produce Vitamin D from exposure to sunlight and to absorb calcium and Vitamin D decreases with age. Getting enough Vitamin D helps the body absorb calcium and also helps the kidneys break down and incorporate (reabsorb) calcium that would otherwise be excreted.

Vitamin D is found in eggs; butter; fatty fish and fortified foods such as milk, orange juice, and cereal. In addition to Vitamin D, a host of other vitamins assist in absorbing calcium and increasing bone mass. They include: Vitamins C, E and K; magnesium, and boron.

Bear in mind: more than 90% of a person's bone mass develops before age 20 years, and half of that bone mass develops from age 11-15 years. Rapid bone loss, however, occurs after age 50. To reduce your risk of osteoporosis, calcium intake should be highest during adolescence and after age 50.

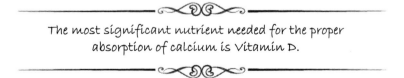

The most significant nutrient needed for the proper absorption of calcium is Vitamin D.

ARE YOU READY TO GO ORGANIC?

Organic food choices fill supermarket shelves – and not just at Whole Foods and other natural food stores where you would expect to find them. Even Wal-Mart now offers organic selections. Many people happily cough up the price – sometimes double – whereas others gaffaw. Who's right? It depends.

 Is organic food really healthier than conventional food?

> The debate about whether organic produce is more nutritious than conventional produce has been around for decades and unfortunately there is currently not sufficient reliable data to definitively and confidently answer this question.
>
> In the meantime there does seem to be compelling intuitive evidence to eat organic and even if the nutritional value isn't one of them, there are many other reasons to buy organic foods. Consider these:
>
> - Absence of pesticide residue.
> - Absence of hormones in food.
> - Absence of antibiotics in food.
> - Animal welfare.
> - Environmental protection.

These are important factors because when we eat non-organic food, we absorb the chemicals and pesticides used on the produce and the hormones and antibiotics given to animals. These substances which are toxic are stored in our cells and as they accumulate over time, they increase our risk of health issues.

Today, you also have to eat more fruit and vegetables to make up for the deficiency of nutrients in these products as a result of agri-business practices: growing food for long shelf-life and cold storage. This means eating more calories and unfortunately a greater consumption of non-organic food also means eating more chemicals.

To help protect yourself here are some basic food preparation practices which can reduce your exposure to pesticide residues on fresh fruits and vegetable:

- Wash produce well to remove bacteria, dirt, waxes and pesticides residues on the surface of foods.
- Peel outer leaves and skin.
- Eat a variety of foods to prevent over-exposure to any one chemical.

A more palatable alternative is to go organic. Or at least pay attention to lists like the one on the next page that provides information about which fruits and vegetables have the highest and lowest pesticide levels. Then try and limit your consumption of those with the highest levels.

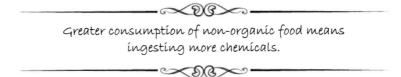

*Greater consumption of non-organic food means
ingesting more chemicals.*

◯ Dirty Dozen™ and Clean 15™ List

The Environmental Working Group (EWG) conducted a study to see which fruits and vegetables had the highest and lowest levels of pesticides. Here's what they found[28]:

Dirty-Dozen™ In other words, try to buy these organic	Clean 15™ Lowest in pesticides, probably don't need to buy organic
1 Apples	1 Onions
2 Celery	2 Sweet Corn
3 Strawberries	3 Pineapples
4 Peaches	4 Avocado
5 Spinach	5 Asparagus
6 Nectarines -imported	6 Sweet peas
7 Grapes - imported	7 Mangoes
8 Sweet bell peppers	8 Eggplant
9 Potatoes	9 Cantaloupe – domestic
10 Blueberries – domestic	10 Kiwi
11 Lettuce	11 Cabbage
12 Kale/collard greens	12 Watermelon
	13 Sweet potatoes
	14 Grapefruit
	15 Mushrooms

◯ Organic Seal of Approval

When buying organic, look for the 100% Organic symbol. To get the USDA organic seal, foods need to have been grown, handled and processed by certified organic facilities. These facilities must be wholly organic.

Meat, poultry, eggs and dairy products need to be produced from animals that have never been given antibiotics or hormones and who have been fed organic crops.

Organic crops must be grown free of conventional pesticides and fertilizers made with synthetic ingredients or sewage sludge, and without bioengineering or use of ionizing radiation.

The USDA is careful to note, however, that an organic seal does not mean a food is healthier or safer than its conventionally grown equivalent. Still, if you prefer not to eat animals fed on sewage sludge, check your area to find out about Organic Food Delivery services which can also save time.

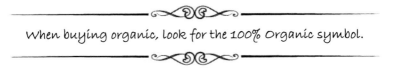

When buying organic, look for the 100% Organic symbol.

Locavore

If you are unable to buy organic produce, try and buy local and seasonal produce. Generally, locally produced items will have a higher nutritional content for obvious reasons: they're picked closer to peak ripeness, and don't have to be in transit or in storage for as long a time.

What's healthy for you is healthy for our planet. Consider also the extraordinary amount of resources that go into shipping a crop from halfway around the world to your local grocery store. Instead, support your local farmer's market – or plant your own fruits and vegetables. As important as whether the food is organic is whether it uses natural resources wisely, relying less on toxic compounds and more on sustainable farming.

Organic? GMO? Or Conventional?

How do you know if your fruits and vegetables are organic, GMO (means genetically modified organism) or conventionally grown (the latter implying regular farming methods using pesticides and herbicides).

Genetically modified means that the genetic material of the substance has been altered by scientists. Is the process or the resulting item then harmful? The jury has yet to decide.

Look at the PLU number or Price Look Up number:

- **If the PLU is a 5-digit number beginning with 9, the item is organic.**
- **If it's a 5-digit number beginning with 8, it's GMO.**
- **If it's a 4-digit number beginning with 4, it's conventionally grown.**

For local produce, check local listings for information on farmers markets in your area. There are bound to be at least a few close by, giving you the opportunity to support local farmers and eat seasonally as well.

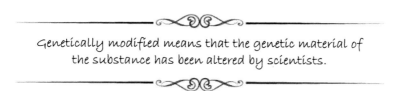

Genetically modified means that the genetic material of the substance has been altered by scientists.

ARE YOU READY TO GO VEGETARIAN?

> "Nothing will benefit human health and increase the
> chances for survival of life on earth as much as the
> evolution to a vegetarian diet."
> ~Albert Einstein. Scientist, Humanitarian

People become vegetarian for many reasons, among them:
ethical, religious, health, a love of animals or even a love of
fads. However, becoming vegetarian while remaining healthy is
not as simple as eliminating animal products.

Vegetarians come in all sorts of denominations:

- **Lacto-ovo vegetarians** do not eat meat, fish or poultry.
- **Lacto vegetarians** do not eat meat, fish, poultry and eggs.
- **Ovo vegetarians** do not eat meat, fish, poultry, milk and
  milk products.
- **Vegans** do not eat any foods of animal origin.
- **Semi vegetarians** are occasional meat eaters.
- **Pesco vegetarians** include fish.
- **Pollo vegetarians** include poultry.

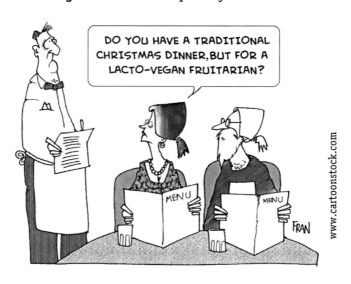

DO YOU HAVE A TRADITIONAL
CHRISTMAS DINNER, BUT FOR A
LACTO-VEGAN FRUITARIAN?

www.cartoonstock.com

Regardless of the type, all vegetarian diets emphasize consumption of the following:

- **Whole grains** – contain protein, are low in fat, provide iron, zinc and B vitamins, and form the basis of a vegetarian diet by contributing calories for energy.

- **Fruits and vegetables** – are a source of essential antioxidants, vitamins, minerals and enzymes.

- **Legumes** (beans, peas and lentils) – are a concentrated plant protein, contain iron, zinc, calcium, Vitamin B6 and fibre.

- **Raw nuts and seeds** – are rich in essential oils.

Now, study the following vegetarian sources of the various macro and micronutrients you'll require.

Protein: Beans, legumes, nuts and seeds need to be combined with rice or other grains to get the essential amino acids needed for optimal health. Hemp, quinoa , soy (tofu, tempeh) and spirulina are the only complete sources of plant protein.

Calcium: **Vegetables sources** are ample but you need a whole bunch mixed with other fortified sources. Vegetable sources include: broccoli, collard greens, dandelion greens, kale, parsley, raw spinach, asparagus, kelp, dulse, okra, tomatoes and green snap peas.

Fruit sources of calcium include: dried figs; prunes; raisins; dates and oranges.

Legume sources include soybeans, cooked dried peas and beans.

Nut and seed sources include almonds, sesame seeds, tahini (crushed sesame seed paste or butter), and walnuts.

Grain sources are amaranth, wheat bran, wheat germ and oats.

Miscellaneous sources include blackstrap molasses, carob, fortified rice beverages, fortified orange juice, whey and yogurt.

Iron: Lentils, garbanzo beans, sesame seeds, almonds, blackstrap molasses, dark leafy, greens, prunes, figs, raisins, dark-green leafy vegetables, strawberries, potatoes, and watermelon are good sources of both Vitamin C and iron. Vitamin C helps increase the absorption of iron from plant foods. You can also get iron by doing some of your cooking in cast iron pots.

B12:   Sea vegetables (dulse and kombu) and natural yogurt. Vitamin B12 is especially important for vegans since it's generally lacking in plant food. Many vegans eat foods fortified with B12 or they take a B12 supplement. Consult with your practitioner.

Omega-3:   Green leafy plants, (dark green leafy vegetables, broccoli), seaweeds, selected seeds (flax, hemp, chia, sacha inchi), nuts (walnuts), soybeans, Omega-3 eggs, and oil extracted from these foods. Note: it is uncertain as to how much EPA and DHA vegans can absorb from plant sources. If your vegan diet is generally sound, you can still be healthy but if you're a strict vegan for the long haul, best to consult with your practitioner.

Omega-6:   Seeds (hemp, pumpkin, sesame, and sunflower), nuts (walnuts), soybeans, and oil extracted from these foods.

ARE YOU READY TO CHANGE YOUR pH?

A healthy vegetarian diet can also help to maintain an overall alkaline state in your body, which is essential for cellular and overall health. **Your body functions best in an alkaline state** (except for inside the stomach, which is acidic).

Regardless of what food we eat, the body has a built-in survival mechanism that keeps it in an alkaline state. However, if we eat too many acidic foods and not enough alkaline ones, the body has to use its own buffers (alkalizing minerals) to neutralize the acidic load. Eating alkaline foods reduces the stress on the body to remain in the proper pH state. Disease thrives in an acidic environment.

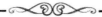

A healthy vegetarian diet can also help to maintain an overall alkaline state in your body, which is essential for cellular and overall health.

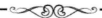

Unfortunately the typical North American diet is very acidic-forming. Not surprisingly, despite our affluence, North Americans have a high rate of contracting many diseases. Our international health profile is no longer so healthy. Obesity and poor diet are the key culprits. Many of the foods that contribute to obesity – ice cream, cake, fatty meats – are acidic.

What is body pH?

The abbreviation pH stands for hydrogen potential, which is a measure of the concentration of hydrogen ions in a solution, or, in other words, a measure of the substance's acidity or alkalinity.

A pH of 7 indicates a neutral solution; a pH below 7 indicates acidity, and a pH in excess of 7 indicates alkalinity.

Your pH level influences weight loss and body fat as well as every biochemical process in your body. For your body to maintain pH balance, it stores a certain amount of excess acid in your fat cells. When a person with a low pH (high acidity) burns fat, the procedure releases the acid that is stored in the person's body fat, thereby potentially putting that person's blood pH out of balance. **Ideally, your pH should be between 7.3 and 7.4 at all times.**

A pH of 7 indicates a neutral solution.
A pH below 7 indicates acidity.
A pH in excess of 7 indicates alkalinity.
Ideally, your pH should be between 7.3 and 7.4 at all times.

pH and Diet

To Maintain Health: our diet should consist of 60% alkaline forming foods and 40% acid forming foods. If you eat largely vegetables – the 40% of acid forming foods in your diet will come from the protein you eat – even beans and legumes are acidic – and grains – which are also acidic.

Most fruits are alkaline. Very few fruits are acidic; cranberries and prunes are an exception. Ironically, oranges, limes and grapefruit are all alkaline. Whether a food contributes to a high or low pH in the body has nothing to do with the acidity of the food outside our body, which is why lemons are alkaline but plums, surprisingly, are acidic forming foods.

To Restore Health: your diet should consist of even more alkaline forming foods – 80% – and fewer acid forming foods – 20%. The Change4Good Program recommends eating vegetables at every meal. Vegetables, of course, are generally alkaline forming.

Although sources vary on the degrees to which certain foods are acid or alkaline forming, below is a general list of foods that tend to be one or the other – once they are digested and absorbed by the body.

Acidic Forming Foods	Sugar, refined salt, condiments such as pickles and ketchup, soda, meat, fish, poultry, eggs, dairy, grains, beans and legumes, fats and oils and some fruits. As you can see, many of the foods we eat are acid-producing. For this reason, it's wise to limit your acid producing quota to foods you really need that supply other nutrients: beans, grains, health fats and healthy fruits. Even putting aside the issue of calories, junk foods are a luxury.
Alkaline Forming Foods	High-water concentrated vegetables such as cucumbers and tomatoes (another food you'd think was acidic); most fruits, root vegetables (potatoes, yams, rutabaga, winter squash), spices, herbs and seasonings, most seeds and nuts, tempeh, whey protein, oriental vegetables, herbal teas and stevia.

Measuring your bodies pH level will determine if your body is alkaline or acidic. You can monitor your pH by checking the pH of your urine or saliva. All you need is pH paper with a range of 5.5-8.5, with small gradient changes. pH paper is sold at your local health food store or pharmacy.

To test your urine:

Collect your first urine of the morning – ideally midstream and in a paper cup. Do not drink any liquids prior to collecting and make sure you collect after at least 6 hours of sleep.

Spot pH paper with drops of urine (see instructions on pH paper package). Compare the colour of the paper with the color chart that comes with the pH paper. Mark this down.

Collect your afternoon and evening urine two hours after a meal. Ideally, you should take your pH reading three times daily. Take all three readings daily for at least three to four weeks.

If you have normal sleeping hours, **the ideal pH range for your urine should be as follows:**

> 7 am   6.6 – 7.0
> 3 pm   6.8 – 7.2
> 9 pm   7.0 – 7.4

To test your saliva:

Upon rising and before drinking any liquids or brushing your teeth, accumulate saliva in your mouth and then discharge the saliva into a spoon or small paper cup. Put the pH paper into the saliva for five to 10 seconds, and then compare the pH with the color chart that comes with the pH paper. Record the results.

The normal pH of saliva is 6.5.

"My refusing to eat meat occasioned inconveniency, and I have been frequently chided for my singularity. But my light repast allows for greater progress, for greater clearness of head and quicker comprehension."

~Benjamin Franklin, 18th Century American Statesman, Inventor

Super Foods

We've covered a lot of different ways in which foods affect our overall health. Confused? You should be. The subject of nutrition – like life itself – is complex. A food that might be helpful from one point of view might not be from another. And of course we're all different and have different priorities. Beware therefore of simple answers or easy generalizations.

Still, some ways of eating – we know – are more helpful than others. Similarly, some foods endure at the top of everyone's "super foods" list despite fluctuations. Therefore, to help you out, here's a list of the Change4Good Top 30 Super Foods©, but of course it doesn't list all of them.

Overall, these foods will help in specific ways to improve muscle building, brain function, cardiovascular health, bone health, immune function and inflammation reduction, wrinkle erasing and some of course, alkalinize your body. Try and incorporate three new super foods into your diet every week.

Super foods help in specific ways to achieve optimal health.

Change4Good Top 30 Super Foods©:

Food	Nutrient	Function
Acai berries	Antioxidants	Protects overall health.
Almonds	Plant sterols, amino acids, Vitamin E	Lowers LDL, lowers blood sugar, muscle growth, free radical protection.
Artichokes	Magnesium, potassium, antioxidants, Vitamin C	Bone health, reduces risk of stroke, immune system health.
Avocado	Monounsaturated fats, folate	Lowers LDL, lowers homocysteine which hinders blood flow through blood vessels.
Black Beans	Anthocyanin, protein, folate, magnesium, B vitamins, potassium	Improves heart health, brain function.
Blueberries	Fibre, Vitamin A and C, antioxidants	Helps prevent a range of diseases from cancer to heart disease.
Bok Choy	Calcium, Vitamin A and C, folic acid, iron	Bone building, lowers blood pressure.
Broccoli	Calcium, manganese, potassium, magnesium, iron, sulforaphane (phytonutrient)	Anti-cancer properties.
Chili Peppers	Beta carotene, capsicin	Stimulates metabolism, natural blood thinner, releases endorphins.
Cinnamon	Antioxidants	Inhibits blood clotting and bacterial growth, stabilizes blood sugar levels.
Dark Chocolate	Flavonoids, procyanidin	Improves blood flow to the brain, keeps arteries flexible and blood pressure low.

Change4Good Top 30 Super Foods©:

Food	Nutrient	Function
Eggs	Protein, minerals	Keeps you satiated and aids with weight loss.
Extra Virgin Olive Oil	Monounsaturated fats, polyphenols	Reduces inflammation in cells and joints.
Figs	Potassium, manganese, antioxidants, fibre	Supports proper pH levels, lowers insulin and blood sugar levels.
Flaxseeds	Protein, fibre, Omega 3	Erases spots and fines lines in the skin, lowers cholesterol.
Ginger	Gingerol	Reduces risk of most cancers.
Green Tea	Catechin (antioxidant)	Anti-inflammatory and anti-cancer properties.
Kiwi	Potassium, Vitamin C, lutein	Bone health, reduces risk of heart disease.
Leeks	Thiamine, riboflavin, calcium, potassium, folic acid	Bone health, lowers homocysteine.
Pineapple	Vitamins, antioxidants, enzymes (bromelain)	Anti-inflammatory, protects against colon cancer and arthritis.
Pomegranates	Polyphenols	Reduces risk of most cancers.
Spinach	Potassium, magnesium, lutein	Muscle builder, prevents clogged arteries, boosts bone-mineral density, reduce risk of certain cancers.
Sweet Potatoes	Glutathione, Vitamin C	Enhances nutrient metabolism and immune system health, helps prevent diabetes, stimulates collagen production.
Tomatoes	Lycopene	Decrease risk of many cancers, eliminate skin aging free radicals from ultraviolet rays.

Change4Good Top 30 Super Foods©:

Food	Nutrient	Function
Tumeric	Curcumin (polyphenol)	Anti-cancer properties, anti-inflammatory effects, decreases amyloid plaques which may cause Alzheimer's disease.
Walnuts	Omega-3, polyphenols, protein	Anti-inflammatory, muscle building, heart health.
Whole Grains	Fibre, protein	Reduces inflammation, keeps colon healthy, fuels brain.
Wild Salmon	Omega-3	Improves nerve communication in brain, metabolism.
Yogurt	Probiotics	Keeps digestive tract healthy, protects immune system.

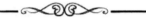

Don't forget your friend water.
Drink the best quality you can find, and drink it
before you even feel the need.

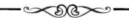

CHANGE4GOOD – ACTION STEPS

- Start implementing Principle 9 – Drink: 1-2 litres of water every day.
- Complete the Change4Good Progress Checklist©.
- Go vegan for one day. You can eat any vegetable, fruit, bean/legume, whole grain, nuts/seeds - eliminate meat, fish, eggs and dairy.
- Monitor your pH balance for one week.
- Identify and complete your eighth short-term (weekly) goal. For example: "I will start drinking warm water with lemon every day; I will include at least one super food in my diet every day; I will find where the local organic food markets are in my area; I will collect at least 3 vegetarian recipes to try."
- Update Change4Good Journal© daily.
- Update Change4Good Goal Sheet© weekly.

TOOLS

- Change4Good Goal Sheet©
- Change4Good Journal©
- Change4Good Progress Checklist©
- Change4Good One Week Cleanse©
- Change4Good Supplement List©
- Change4Good Top 30 Super Foods List©

REMEMBER THIS

- The joy of eating also includes doing what's good for your health and our planet.

Change Your Fitness

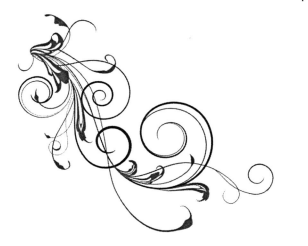

Chapter TEN

REV UP YOUR METABOLISM (BUT SANELY)

This chapter is about turning all those nutrients into energy; it's about, having every muscle in your body shout, "Rah!"

Principle **10** Move: Exercise at Least 30-60 Minutes Every Day

Physical activity burns calories, increases metabolic rate and energy, and relieves stress. In other words, it's a win-win situation. You feel better; you look great.

"There are really only two requirements when it comes to exercise. One is that you do it. The other is that you continue to do it."
~The New Glucose Revolution for Diabetes by Jennie Brand-Miller, Kaye Foster-Powell, Stephen Colagiuri and Alan W. Barclay

Ever wonder why some people can eat and eat and never gain a pound while you seem to gain weight just looking at food? Or why a man who goes on the same diet as a woman loses more weight more quickly – even cheating? The answer is in part, your food and beverage intake and physical activity level, but also your metabolism.

Your metabolism is what determines how much total energy or calories your body needs on a daily basis, not just to support all the activities you do, but also to sustain itself at rest. In other words, the energy (from food and beverages) it needs to support all the biochemical reactions that occur within our cells, to maintain amongst many other things, a normal body temperature, circulate blood, repair cells, breathe, etc.

The number of calories your body uses to perform these basic functions is known as your basal or resting metabolic rate or metabolism. These energy needs remain fairly consistent and generally account for about 60-75% of the calories you burn every day. As we know, metabolic rates differ and a fast, efficient metabolism can consume a lot of calories. A slower metabolism consumes fewer calories. The calories or energy we don't use get sored as fat cells for later use. To lose one pound of body fat, a person must "burn" 3500 calories.

What Affects Metabolism?

Several factors affect your basal metabolic rate and how many calories you burn each day:

- Food metabolism (thermogenesis/thermic effect of food) including digestion, absorption, transport and storing all require calories. This accounts for about 10% of your total daily energy expenditure or calories used each day. Here we will see that a calorie is not just a calorie. Different macronutrients require more or fewer calories to metabolize or break them down so that they can be used as fuel.

- Body Composition and Size.
- Hormones and Stress.
- Age.
- Gender.
- Physical Activity accounts for the rest of the calories your body burns each day, approximately 30% of your total daily energy expenditure. Obviously, the more strenuous the exercise, the more calories burned.

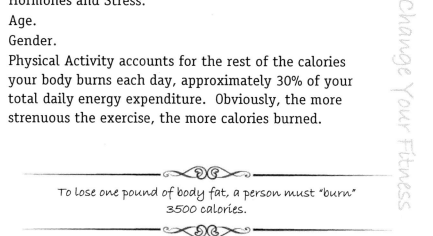

To lose one pound of body fat, a person must "burn" 3500 calories.

Before looking at the significant role of exercise in boosting metabolism, let's look at all the other sources of influence in greater detail, beginning with the one with which we're most familiar.

1. FOOD

Let's begin our discussion with the thermic effect of food. This is the amount of energy required to metabolize a particular food. A calorie is not just a calorie. **Different macronutrients require more or fewer calories to metabolize or break them down so that they can be used as fuel.**

For example, your body uses approximately:

- 30% of calories to metabolize protein.
- 8-9% of calories to metabolize carbohydrates.
- 3% of calories to metabolize fat.

More calories remain to be stored as fat from a carbohydrate or fat-laden meal than a protein-dense one. Here is an example to illustrate the thermic effect of food:

Meal A (High Carbohydrate)			Meal B (High Protein)		
10g Protein	30g Carbohydrate	10g Fat	30g Protein	10g Carbohydrate	10g Fat
1 chicken thigh (10g protein)			3.5 oz chicken breast (30g protein)		
1 ½ cups green peas (30g carbohydrate)			½ cup green peas (10g carbohydrate)		
2 tsp olive oil (10g fat)			2 tsp olive oil (10g fat)		
Total calories consumed: 250			Total calories consumed: 250 (same as Meal A)		
Total calories used to metabolize the meal: 22.			Total calories used to metabolize the meal: 41. (19 more calories than for Meal A)		

The thermic effect from a protein meal compared to a high carbohydrate or fat meal is greater – this is one of the scientific underpinnings for why you should follow Principle 4 which tells you to include protein at every meal. It also fills us up and further delays hunger. Additionally, protein is essential for building and repairing muscle tissue, particularly in response to exercise.

Certain items like cayenne and hot peppers are also said to increase metabolic rate, but the impact of these foods is truly minimal.

Unfortunately, the typical North American diet today consists of a high amount of refined and processed carbohydrates – white rice, pasta, bread, pastries, candy, cereals and other flour and sugar-laden foods and beverages.

Such foods are quickly broken down by the body, which, as we have seen in Chapter FOUR, causes an insulin spike. You recall that when carbohydrates are broken down into sugar (glucose), the body releases insulin in order to clear the glucose from the bloodstream. The more refined carbohydrates are broken down quickly, enter the bloodstream quicker and therefore cause a greater and faster release of insulin.

How does this relate to metabolism?

High levels of insulin both in the blood and cells create a sluggish metabolism. Biochemically, high insulin levels reduce the levels of a hormone-sensitive, fat-releasing enzyme called lipo-protein lipase.

Conversely, low insulin levels increase the levels of glucagons, which mobilize fat so that the enzyme carriers can transport them into the muscle cells for use as fuel. Remember the glycemic cycle:

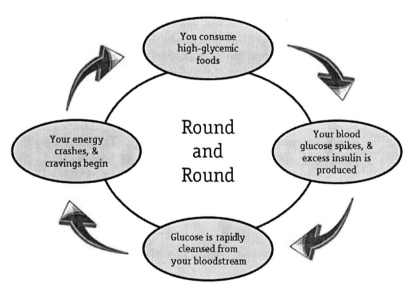

The good news: you can keep insulin levels low by changing your diet, and exercising properly following the 10 Change4Good Principles©.

Let's look in more detail at fats as well. Essential fats (EFAs), namely Omega-3 and Omega-6 fats, supply the building blocks of various structures in the body; including cell membranes. These fats also work together to increase the overall amount of oxygen utilized by the cells to produce energy. The more oxygen we transport to our cells, the faster we burn body fat. EFAs also increase insulin efficiency of the body.

Additionally, as mentioned in Chapter FOUR, although EFAs improve metabolic health, findings are inconclusive as to whether they play a significant role in actually stimulating fat burning.

Water is also critical for fat burning. There are numerous theories as to how water affects metabolism. What we know for sure is that proper hydration and, in particular, proper cell hydration is essential for optimal cell functioning and therefore also fat metabolism. Even being mildly dehydrated can slow your metabolism by as much as 3%.

Other factors come into play as well. Theoretically if we eat fewer calories than we use, we should lose weight, right? Not entirely. In fact, **consuming too few calories slows our metabolic rate.** To avoid starvation, the body, struggling to conserve energy, burns fewer calories.

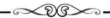

The smartest strategy for healthy weight loss is to consume the greatest number of calories that will allow you to still lose weight – rather than the lowest number.

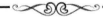

Another factor is the effect of eating frequency on metabolism. It has long been believed that **eating frequent meals/snacks throughout the day increases or at least maintains our resting metabolic rate.**

The rationale and some science reveals that when you have not eaten for a long period of time, your metabolism will be functioning at a lower capacity as your body senses itself going into starvation mode. When you do eventually eat, your metabolism is not as well equipped to utilize the food and much of it will therefore be stored as body fat. In addition, your body also stores this food in anticipation of a possible future "starvation" period.

This is similar to what would happen if you were to start a fire by simply throwing down a big log and holding a match to it - the log would take forever to burn, if at all. Instead, you use paper and small pieces of kindling. Together with the paper, the kindling starts a small flame and more heat is generated. When the flame gets larger, you add larger pieces of wood until the fire is blazing hot and then as you continue to add fuel to the fire, it maintains its heat, just as your metabolism would.

A recent review of scientific literature on eating frequency published in the *Journal of the International Society of Sports Nutrition*, states that although eating frequency does not appear to favourably change body composition in sedentary people, it does help decrease hunger and improves appetite control.[29]

Regardless of the effect of *eating frequency* on body composition, we know for sure that eating 4-6 small nutrient dense meals/snacks (Principle 4) increases metabolism, even if only slightly, thanks to the thermic effect of food.

To recap, your body has to work (burn calories) to digest, absorb and process nutrients. Each time you eat, body temperature increases slightly and that increases your metabolism. In addition, eating frequently prevents us from getting overly hungry and therefore overeating. It also prevents our blood sugar levels from crashing and causing mood swings and cravings for sugary foods – none of which are healthy.

For these reasons, you should not only eat 4-6 small meals/snacks throughout the day (divide lunch into a sandwich and fruit that you'll eat as a snack later) but include protein in most of them.

However, eating more calories than you require produces fat cells, and fat cells don't go away on their own. Once you have one, it's yours for life. So this is why you also need to monitor the portions of those 4-6 small meals/snacks (Principle 7).

So in conclusion, follow the Change4Good Principles© and eat correct portions of food, with a balance of nutrient-dense lean protein, natural carbohydrates and healthy fats regularly throughout the day, while drinking enough water. This is the most efficient way to achieve and maintain a healthy weight.

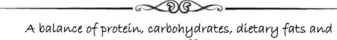

A balance of protein, carbohydrates, dietary fats and water proves to be the most efficient way to maintain a healthy weight.

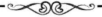

BODY COMPOSITION

Body composition is the relationship between lean mass to fat mass. Lean mass includes the non-fat tissues such as bones, tendons, ligaments, organs, muscle and fluids.

Obviously, you'll look better with more lean muscle mass than fat. But you'll also burn more calories. Muscle is more metabolically active than fat, and muscle is the prime site for burning fat. The more muscle you have, the more fat you can burn for energy.

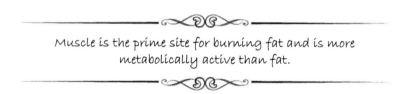

Muscle is the prime site for burning fat and is more
metabolically active than fat.

One pound of muscle burns about ten calories per day; a pound of fat burns only about three calories per day. Therefore, by losing muscle tissue we are slowing our metabolism. Increasing muscle tissue increases metabolism. How do you increase muscle tissue? Through strength training – not through eating excessive amounts of protein, as some mistakenly believe.

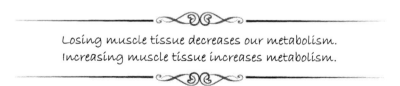

Losing muscle tissue decreases our metabolism.
Increasing muscle tissue increases metabolism.

1. HORMONES and STRESS

Insulin, thyroid hormones, estrogen, testosterone, growth hormone and stress hormones (like cortisol) all have a significant effect on fat, calorie-burning and muscle gain and loss.

Cortisol increases weight gain. How? It is released by the adrenal glands when we are under both real or imagined stress (and who doesn't experience stress on a regular basis). How? It stimulates the production of glucose, which then stimulates insulin. Insulin, in turn, causes glucose to get stored as fat. Cortisol also stimulates our appetite.

Stress and the excess cortisol it produces also makes you feel tired; which causes some people to eat on the erroneous assumption that calories will give them the energy they need. The extra calories, however, only cause weight gain, particularly around the abdomen area. Fat cells in that area are most sensitive to cortisol.

Obviously, it would be better for your body and your mind not to feel stress. But perhaps these palpable consequences of stress will give you even more incentive to chill.

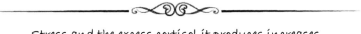

Stress and the excess cortisol it produces increases appetite and causes weight gain, particularly in the abdomen area.

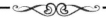

If your relationships unnerve you, detach (for the time being). Sometimes our problem is simply making another person's problem our own. Moderation not perfection is another slogan to emblazon on your brain. Make serenity your goal and other goals (the practical ones) will grace your life in the proper time. Changing your attitude (Chapter ONE) and managing obstacles (Chapter THREE) also helps. In brief: change what you can and work hard to accept the rest.

4. AGE

As **you age, your metabolic rate slows down.** Even super athletes who become less active lose muscle mass. During mid-life, hormones also lessen our rate of fat and calorie burning. However, if you stay active and continue to strength train, you can minimize these effects.

5. GENDER

In case you've ever wondered why your male partner/friend can eat far more than you and lose weight; here's why. **Women naturally have more fat and less muscle than men;** therefore, women's resting metabolic rates are usually lower than those of men who are the same age, height and weight.

6. EXERCISE

> **"Lack of activity destroys the good condition of every human being, while movement and methodical physical exercise save it and preserve it. "**
> ~Plato, Greek Philosopher

Move: Exercise at Least 30-60 Minutes Every Day

From the beginning of time, humans were meant to move. We had to in order to survive. Now, thanks to technology, we don't have to be nearly as active. Our bodies, on the other hand, still need to move in order to function optimally. In addition, physical activity and exercise have the greatest impact on metabolism.

Today the Surgeon General's report warns that physical inactivity is a major health risk. The Center for Disease Control and Prevention says that in addition to genetics, lack of exercise and obesity due to poor nutrition comprises the second-largest cause of death.[30] As a society, we now need to exercise.

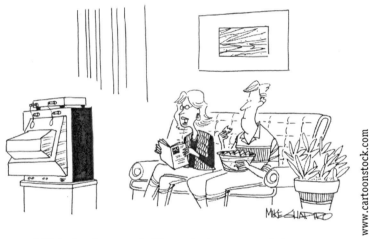

" This looks good. It's a six-hour special on how society is becoming too sedentary."

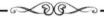

In addition to genetics, lack of exercise and obesity due to poor nutrition comprises the second-largest cause of death.

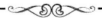

The good news is that whenever you start, the benefits are tremendous. There are hundreds of benefits to exercise, such as:

- **A better ability to cope with stress.**
- **Lower levels of anxiety and depression.**
- **Improved mood** due to the release of endorphins and energy.
- **Better sleep.**
- **Improved self-esteem.**
- **Reduced risk of heart disease, diabetes, high blood pressure, certain cancers and osteoporosis.**
- **Increased muscle strength, flexibility and flow of blood to joints.**
- **A stronger cardiovascular system.**
- **Lower blood sugar levels.**
- **Improved body composition.**
- **Weight loss and maintenance of weight.**

And those are just a few....

Not everyone is born loving to work out. I didn't start out in life loving to go to the gym at 6:30 a.m. As I mentioned in my biography (My Story); my entry into exercise began through sports: I swam and I played competitive tennis. I only became truly interested in fitness as a means to an end when I moved to Canada and, having long given up competitive tennis, I moved into a condo across the street from a gym. Working out was convenient; furthermore, I liked how it made me feel. I started with machines in the gym. When I began to study personal training, I learned about technique. I switched from machines to free weights.

In general, it takes about three to six months to see a real change in your physique. As I reached that point, I could see that my muscles had more definition; my body more shape; my waist was smaller; my arms had firm curves. My glutes, quads and hamstrings had totally changed – those areas of my body had more definition and became thinner. I also liked feeling that I had worked a muscle. I knew when I felt a bit sore the next day that I had strengthened a muscle. My energy increased and best of all, my mood improved.

Eventually, I arrived at the point where I am now. I work hard to stay fit but not nearly as hard as I did to get fit.

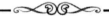

Exercising will supercharge your metabolism, and have the greatest effect on your ability maintain a healthy weight and a lean, toned body.

Just as in nutrition three macronutrients are needed for optimal health, **three components of exercise are essential for optimal fitness:**

- Cardiovascular exercise
- Strength training
- Flexibility

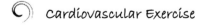 *Cardiovascular Exercise*

Cardiovascular or aerobic exercise is any repetitive movement that uses the large muscle groups of the body for an extended period of time resulting in a sustained increase in heart rate.

It stimulates the cardiovascular, respiratory and circulatory systems. It also allows you to burn calories primarily from fat and carbohydrates. Examples of good cardiovascular exercises are: walking (at more than a leisurely pace), jogging, swimming, cycling, rollerblading, cross-country skiing and taking fast-paced aerobics classes.

Strength Training

Strength training uses resistance to overload the muscles and thereby increase muscle mass, strength and endurance. In increasing strength, it helps reduce the risk of injury; it also increases bone mass and helps to increase and maintain muscle mass.

From a weight management perspective, strength training is critical.

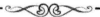

After age 30, everyone loses about half a pound of muscle each year unless they strength train.

If you weighed 120 pounds at age 20 and you weigh the same now at age 40, you've replaced up to 10 pounds of muscle with 10 pounds of fat (unless you've been regularly strength training).

Increased muscle mass is essential for metabolism and a healthy body composition. In terms of equipment, strength training utilizes first and foremost your own body weight, and in addition, equipment such as dumbbells, strength-training machines, and resistance bands.

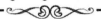

*Increased muscle mass is essential for metabolism and
a healthy body composition.*

Flexibility

Flexibility is often the most neglected component of fitness. It involves gentle, controlled exercises that help increase the range of motion of our body's joints.

Flexibility training helps maintain our overall mobility (especially as we age) and also helps to reduce exercise-related injuries. Examples include yoga or merely stretches during or after each strength training workout and after each cardio workout.

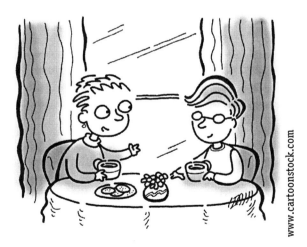

www.cartoonstock.com

"I find yoga very relaxing. Until the
kids get back from yoga class."

Change4Good Fitness GPS©

Now that you are aware of the basic components required for optimal fitness, you're ready to complete your Fitness GPS.

Below is an example of a completed Change4Good Fitness GPS©.

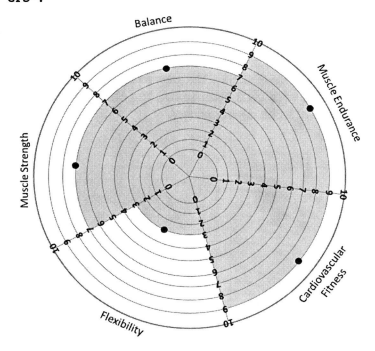

For your own purposes, either use the blank Change4Good Fitness GPS© on the next page or download it at **www.change4good.ca.**

Your Change4Good Fitness GPS©

What to do:

1. Using the Change4Good Fitness GPS© rate your level of satisfaction for each separate area between zero and ten (ten being complete satisfaction; zero being none).

2. Place one dot (per segment) opposite the number that best represents your level of satisfaction.

3. Connect the dots to create a "circle" within the Change4Good Fitness GPS©. **Unless you're equally satisfied or dissatisfied with each component, the circle-within-the-circle is bound to be *asymmetrical*.**

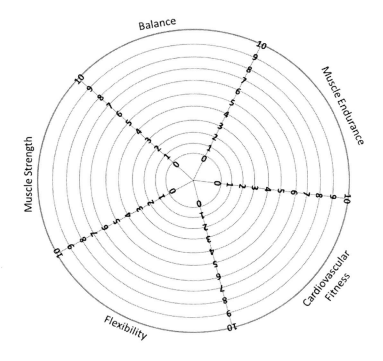

Now consider the following:

1. **How large is your circle?** Bigger is better.
2. **How symmetrical is it?** Your goal is to push everything to the outer rim, to have the largest, roundest circle.
3. **Where does your circle dip toward the center? The dips indicate the areas you most need to address.** Use the information below to guide you in developing your program. Always consult with your health provider before starting an exercise program. Hire a qualified and experienced trainer, at least initially, to ensure that your program is safe and appropriate.

FITT Program for Exercise

In the acronym **FITT**, the letters stand for:
Frequency, **I**ntensity, **T**ime and **T**ype.

This is a basic formula to ensure you are covering all the necessary components of an exercise program. Apply the FITT guidelines to cardiovascular, strength and flexibility training. Below are recommendations for the three essential components of a balanced exercise program.

Caveats: Do not forget to warm-up and cool-down which is discussed further along in the chapter. Start a bit slower and build – it will increase your pleasure and reduce your risk of injury. If you have been sedentary, don't aim for six days per week. If you are already doing three days per week, consider increasing to 5 or 6 days per week.

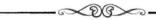

Do not forget to warm-up and cool-down. Start a bit slower and build – it will increase your pleasure and reduce your risk of injury.

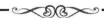

◯ . Frequency: **The number of times per week you should workout**

1. **Cardiovascular Training: 3-5+ days per week.**
2. **Strength Training: 2-3 days per week for major muscle groups.**

   Do 2-3 days if you work all major muscle groups in one workout; four days if you do a split program such as upper body one day and lower body the next. You want to work each of the major muscle groups at least twice per week but never on consecutive days in order to allow muscles to recover.

   Major muscle groups are:
   - Chest
   - Back
   - Biceps (front muscles of upper arm)
   - Triceps (muscles of back upper arm)
   - Shoulders
   - Quadriceps (front of thigh)
   - Hamstrings (back of thigh)
   - Glutes (butt)
   - Core (muscles that link upper and lower extremities, the major muscles being the abdominals in the area between the mid and lower back)

3. **Flexibility Training: every day that you exercise, but at least 2-3 days per week.**

Intensity: **How hard you should workout or, your exertion level**

1. **Cardiovascular Training**

   Here we use the term **target heart rate** (THR), **which is the recommended heart rate zone or intensity at which you should be working.** The goal is to raise your resting heart rate to a specific range in order to gain an aerobic benefit.

   To determine your THR:

   - First determine your maximum heart rate by subtracting your age from 220. For example, if you are 30 years old, your maximum heart rate is 220 minus 30, or 190.
   - Next, multiply 190 by **65%** (or multiply 190 by 65 and then divide by 100). That number represents the **low end** of your range.
   - Now multiply the same 190 by **85%** (or multiply 190 by 85 and then divide by 100). The result will be the **high range.**
   - For someone 30 years old, then, the target heart rate is 123.5-161.5 heartbeats per minute.
   - Or, to make THR easier to monitor, divide the final answer by 6, which gives you the number of beats per 10 seconds.

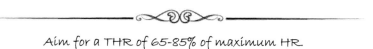

Aim for a THR of 65-85% of maximum HR.

Easier methods are to use a heart rate monitor, which you can buy, or monitor your exertion based simply on how you feel. **The latter is commonly referred to as Rating of Perceived Exertion.** My clients use a scale from 1–10, with 1 representing no effort (a walk in the park) and 10, the maximum (Everest climbing).

Aim to work out at a level between 6.5 **(which should feel like you are rushing to an appointment that you are late for)-8.5 (which should feel as if you are working out at an intensity that you are not sure you can maintain for approximately 45 minutes but you probably could).**

Another easy method to measure THR is the **Talk Test.** See how well you can converse while you work. If you are only able to utter a couple of words and not full sentences then you know you are probably working at the right level of intensity for you.

You can also monitor your overall increase in fitness by monitoring your resting heart rate (take your pulse first thing in the morning before you get out of bed). The fitter you get the lower this number will be. **A typical resting heart for adults is 60–100 beats per minute.** However conditioned athletes and people doing regular exercise often have resting heart rates between 40 and 60 beats per minutes.

Another gauge is how quickly you recover after a workout – the quicker you return to your resting heart rate after your workout the fitter you are becoming.

2. Strength Training

In strength training, intensity is determined by the amount of weight lifted and the numbers of both repetitions (reps) and sets of repetitions performed. Regardless of the number of sets and reps you do, choose a weight that will take you to muscle failure by the last few reps – muscle failure being the point at which you literally could not lift the weight one more time.

Never compromise technique. Best to start with a greater number of reps (approximately 15-20), a lesser weight and 1-2 sets. Then as your muscular endurance improves, you become more fit, and your joints, ligaments and tendons are more conditioned; increase the weight and reduce the number of reps (2-4 sets of 10-15 reps to improve strength and 2-4 sets of 8-12 reps to improve strength and power).

Another way to create intensity in a weight-training workout is to do a strength interval circuit. In this kind of workout, you do as many reps as you can, using a particular weight and working in a fixed amount of time. For example, you could do as many biceps curls as you can in 20 seconds; then rest for 10 seconds; then repeat. The number of times you repeat the lift/rest/lift cycle depends on your fitness level and goals. Again, never compromise weight lifted or speed of exercise for technique.

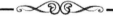

Regardless of the number of sets and reps you do, choose a weight that will take you to muscle failure by the last few reps, but never compromise technique.

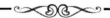

3. **Flexibility**

Stretch to the point that you feel tension but never pain.

🌀 *Time:* **The duration of the workout**

1. **Cardiovascular Training:** 20-60 minutes per session.

The time will depend on the intensity level at which you are working. The higher the intensity or effort expended, the shorter the duration. For example, if I only have 30 minutes in which to run, I am going to have to run at a faster speed in order to get the same benefit from doing a 60 minute run.

2. **Strength Training:** 15-60 minutes.

Here, too, time spent depends on the program.

3. **Flexibility:** Hold each stretch for approximately 30 seconds and repeat 2-4 times.

The total amount of time spent depends on: whether you're doing an entire flexibility class (like yoga) or merely stretching selected muscles.

Caveat: Never stretch before a workout. Your muscles are cold at that point, and at risk of injury. Think of how inflexible an uncooked piece of spaghetti is versus a cooked piece. The uncooked spaghetti is your cold muscle.

Combining these three components aim for an average of 5 hours per week (depending of course on your fitness goals).

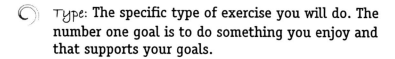

Type: **The specific type of exercise you will do. The number one goal is to do something you enjoy and that supports your goals.**

1. **Cardiovascular Training:**

   Such as walking, swimming, running, cross-country skiing and other sports that significantly increase heart rate.

   The question I am asked most frequently is: what is the best type of cardio to do? My answer: what you enjoy because that is what you will do.

2. **Strength Training:**

   Such as weight training using dumbbells, machines, body weight or resistance bands, even Pilates.

   Ideally, you want to focus on all the major muscle groups. Aim for a variety of types of strength training and exercises.

   - **Multi-joint exercises** are those that involve two or more joints and are preferable as you become more advanced, for example, lunges.
   - **Single joint or isolation exercises** involve a single joint or muscle, for example, seated leg curls.

   When you do a lunge for example, you use almost all the muscles in your body – calves, quadriceps, hamstrings, glutes, core and even the upper body, which you use to maintain proper posture. Balance, too, is required. All these elements come into play, which is, of course, beneficial.

When you do a seated leg curl, however, sitting down with a backrest, you are only engaging the hamstrings. In other words, you're using fewer muscles; the workload is easier; you burn fewer calories, and don't benefit in as many ways as you do when you do lunges.

- **Single joint exercises**, however, may be beneficial for a beginner. They'll help her/him learn proper body positioning and build up base strength, while, at the same time, providing support and stability. If balance is a factor, single joint exercises may be safer. They can also allow injured people to maintain their fitness without harming the afflicted muscle or area. For example, if someone has a sprained ankle, she/he could do seated leg curls and still maintain hamstring strength.

- **Functional exercises** mimic daily activities or a particular sport you play. You may be able to do a chest press with 50lb dumbbells or biceps curls with 20lb dumbbells, but are you able to carry your groceries from the car without pulling out your back?

  Functional exercises are about teaching the muscles to work together; they're about doing exercises in which you have to support your own weight as much as possible. A more functional exercise than a chest press, in this case, would be a push-up or a standing cable chest press. (Unlike a chest press on a bench, in both the latter cases, you're using your leg muscles and core for support). **Ideally, you want to do exercises that simultaneously use different muscles.**

  Caveat: make sure you do all exercises through a full range of motion, that is: the movement from the beginning to the finishing point of the exercise.

3. **Flexibility:** General stretching within or after a workout, or yoga.

Warming Up, Cooling Down

Regardless of the type of workout being done, you always need to warm up and cool down. **The warm up can be anywhere from 5–10 minutes, depending on the length of the workout; the cool down should be about 5 minutes.** Both are critical to preventing injuries. The warm-up prepares the body for the workout to come: gradually increasing heart rate and body temperature; warming up the muscles, and increasing blood and fluid flow to the joints. The cool down gradually brings the body back to its regular resting state.

Two options for the warm up are to do a general activity like walking or using an elliptical trainer or bike – or, to do the same activity that you'll be doing in the workout, but at a lower intensity. For example if I am going to run, my warm-up could be a light jog. For weight training, I might jog on the treadmill or elliptical or I can do my weight-training regimen but first with lighter weights and more reps. If I'm going to do a set of chest press, I'll use lighter weights and do extra reps. The goal, again, is to warm up the muscles, lubricate the joints and prepare the body for the demand you are about to place on it.

To safely cool down at the end of a workout, gradually decrease the exercise intensity to bring the body back to its pre-exercise state.

Remember: flexibility exercises and stretching should only be done when the body and muscles are already warm - either during the workout, between sets or afterwards.

Design Your Regimen: Principles to Bear in Mind

1. Specificity of Training

Train in a specific way to achieve a specific outcome. For example, if I want to train for a 10km running race, I might do some of my training on a bike or elliptical, as well as some weight training for added strength, for the purpose of cross training (see definition below), but not all of it. I'd want my training to predominantly be running.

Cross training involves training in different ways to maintain fitness but reduce the risk of injury. For example if I am a runner, my cross-training could be using an elliptical trainer or cycling. I am still working my cardiovascular system and my legs but I am giving my joints a break from the pounding of running. It also reduces the risk of boredom with training.

Or, if I want to increase my strength, then I need to use heavier weights and do fewer repetitions in order to achieve the desired result. I also need to train the specific areas I wish to strengthen.

The point is: before you design your program, know what goals you want to achieve.

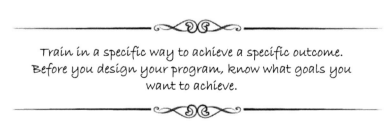

Train in a specific way to achieve a specific outcome. Before you design your program, know what goals you want to achieve.

2. Progressive Overload

As mentioned earlier, **in order to gain fitness you need to overload your body and the muscles above and beyond their comfort zone.** It's the extra stress you put on your body that causes it to strengthen. If I want to be able to run for 45 minutes, for example, but I never run more than 30 minutes, I won't achieve my goal. If I want my biceps to get stronger or larger but I never lift weights that are heavier than what I can do without much effort, my body won't respond by growing muscle.

3. Consistency

As with nutrition, consistency is crucial. It is better to workout three days every week than six days a week for two weeks and then not workout for the next two weeks.

Moderation and consistency, not perfection – that should be your mantra. The only area in which perfection should be your goal is with respect to technique: strive for perfect technique to avoid injury and work the target muscles.

4. Individuality

Everyone's body responds differently to exercise (and nutrition). It's important then to know your body and monitor how it responds to a particular regimen. Monitoring allows you to tweak your program. What works wonders for your friend may not work well for you. Remember Principle 2? It applies to exercise just as it does to nutrition: use an exercise journal (see later in chapter) to track your exercise progress. In addition, just as we did with nutrition, establish particular goals. On the next page is a sample of my weekly exercise regimen. Bear in mind I'm currently on a maintenance fitness program.

Lauren's Week:

Monday	45 minutes of cardio – either running or the elliptical.
Tuesday	My 700 Rep Total Conditioning Circuit (page 336) or Recovery Day.
Wednesday	45 minutes of cardio – either running or the elliptical.
Thursday	A weight training workout focusing on upper body strength.
Friday	Recovery Day.
Saturday	45 minutes of cardio – either running or the elliptical.
Sunday	My 700 Rep Total Conditioning Circuit (page 336).

One of my criteria for buying a condo was to make sure it had a gym. The presence of one right in the complex helps enormously when it's 6:30 a.m. and I don't want to get up. I've been working with weights so long that I know what to do but a newcomer might want to take a minimum of three to five sessions with a personal trainer. Videos are nice but they can't tell you what you're doing wrong.

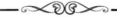

It's important then to know your body and monitor how it responds to a particular regimen. Monitoring allows you to tweak your program.

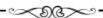

For cardio, as I said, I mostly run or do the elliptical. But my routine varies. In summer, I power walk, run outdoors or use the elliptical. In winter it's primarily the treadmill and stepmill or elliptical. I'll sometimes also swim or cycle. Sometimes I'll take a spinning class. On vacation, I do things I don't get to do at home. If there's a lake nearby, I'll swim. And of course I still play tennis at any opportunity possible.

Be flexible and follow your gut – except when it tells you to skip your routine. Doing it almost always feels better – except when you're injured or truly fatigued.

5. Reversibility

Unfortunately, fitness doesn't last. **The gains you make from training only last if you continue to exercise.** As soon as you stop, you start to lose cardiovascular fitness, strength and flexibility.

We generally lose cardiovascular fitness and flexibility much quicker than strength. The reversibility of fitness affirms the importance of consistency. How quickly you lose the gains you've made depends on your overall fitness level, how long you've been working out and how long you haven't. The shorter the time you have been training for and the longer the time away, the longer it will take you to recoup.

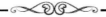

Fitness doesn't last. The gains you make from training only last if you continue to exercise. As soon as you stop, you start to lose cardiovascular fitness, strength and flexibility.

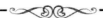

6. Stress/Rest

In order for us to grow more fit, we need to stress our muscles. At the same time, however, we also need to rest.

Resting, the body can repair itself, and strengthen. Our muscle mass can increase. Rest is a valuable part of this process, which is why it is important not to work the same muscle group two days in a row.

The rest part of the equation is just as important as the strength part. Without it, the body can't repair and strengthen and new injuries will forestall future workouts.

Muscles grow and repair when you rest. If you did weight training using the same muscle group every day, you would essentially get weaker as that muscle would never get the rest it needs to repair and strengthen.

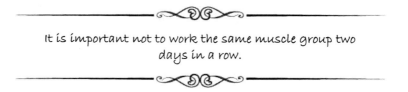

It is important not to work the same muscle group two days in a row.

7. Fun/Enjoyment

Life is full of chores; exercise shouldn't be one of them. Find what you enjoy. **If you enjoy it, you'll do it and if you do it, you'll get results.** If exercise is your time out for solitude, then skip the group sport activities. Search and find what will give you pleasure both physically and emotionally. Like a great relationship, you want to be involved with some kind of exercise routine for the long haul.

Workout Strategies to Jump-Start Your Metabolism and Maximize Results

Before randomly trying any of the following workout concepts, consider your goals and current fitness level. What follows is what has worked for my clients. Remember, because our bodies adapt so quickly, keep changing your routine in order to keep making strides.

1. **High-Intensity Interval and Endurance Training**

    Insert close to maximal-intensity intervals within a moderate intensity workout.

    An example: do repeated 30-second sprints within your regular run. Do not, however, let your super-tough intervals last longer than one to two minutes.

    Another example: do a tougher than usual set for each muscle group within your regular strength training routine. The result in both cases is that you will burn more glycogen, fat and calories.

    Alternatively do higher intensity steady state endurance training.

    For example run for 45 minutes at the maximum intensity that you can sustain for the duration of the run. The benefit, more calories burned both during and after the workout.

    A recent paper in the Medicine and Science in Sports and Exercise Journal showed that when individuals (in this case, males between 22–33 years old) worked out for 45 minutes at a high intensity (70% of VO_2Max which is the maximum amount of oxygen a person's body can use during exercise) they were able to increase the total amount of calories burned by 37% due to the additional calories their bodies continued to burn for 14 hours post exercise.[31]

In addition to burning more total calories and temporarily increasing your resting metabolic rate, **high-intensity interval training increases your fitness level more rapidly than moderate steady-state training.** Ideally, it is best to do a combination of both: shorter, high intensity intervals to maximize fitness gains and improve body composition and longer steady-state workouts, but still at a relatively high intensity to improve your overall endurance capacity. In summary, work as hard as you can for the duration of your training session.

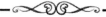

Ideally, it is best to do a combination of shorter, high intensity intervals to maximize fitness gains and improve body composition and longer steady-state workouts to improve overall endurance capacity.

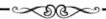

2. Lift Heavier Weights

Women, in particular, run a mile (or ten) when they hear me say this but the reality is, **if you want to improve your body composition, body shape and increase your muscle mass and strength, then you need to lift heavy weights.** Lifting heavier weights tears more muscle s than lighter training. To compensate, the body must work even harder to rebuild that muscle after the workout is over, triggering an immediate post-workout boost.

Endurance athletes, on the other hand, need to develop the energy and neuromuscular systems necessary for endurance activities. In their case, focusing on muscular endurance (greater number of reps) first in the weight training workouts and then progressing into more strength training (lower number of reps) in the off-season makes sense.

Remember, exercise selection should always be specifically tailored to meet your goals – or it should result in exercises that mimic the needs of the endurance activity in which you're engaged.

3. Vary Exercises

If you always use the treadmill, try the bike or elliptical trainer. If you always do the same program on the elliptical, try a different one. Your body gets used to the same routine so that it eventually does not have to burn as many calories as it previously did for the same workout.

Keep your body guessing and burning more calories by changing your cardio workouts regularly. Keep in mind as well that when using a treadmill a grade of 0 is actually slightly downhill and a grade of 1.0 is a flat surface so try and work at least a 2.0 grade to more closely mimic walking or running outdoors.

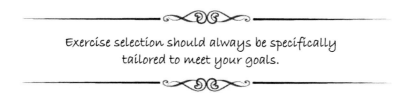

Exercise selection should always be specifically tailored to meet your goals.

For strength training, try a different exercise for every muscle group. When you work your muscles from different angles, you reach different s and stimulate more growth. Instead of doing the same flat-bench dumb-bell chest press, try performing a chest-press on an incline or do push-ups. For each muscle group the possibilities are virtually limitless.

Also, **vary the repetitions and weight lifted per set.** Even just change the order in which you usually do your routine. Keep in mind that the body can begin to adapt to the same routine in as little as six sessions.

Weather permitting, take your workout outdoors. Cultivate the pleasure of being amid nature. The beauty helps alleviate stress and the change of setting relieves boredom – an enemy of consistency. Other benefits of working outdoors:

- You'll have to control of your body more; working out on a natural, possibly uneven surface allows a more thorough activation of joints and muscles.
- You burn more calories due to the higher intensity workout, greater physical demands of unpredictable terrain and the increased mental focus required to stay on track.
- Your body and mind will thank you for this experience.

4. Circuit Train

Circuit training involves moving from one muscle group or exercise to the next during a workout, with as little rest as possible between exercises. Circuit training allows you to burn more calories by working a greater number of muscles in less time. Also, it makes your workout more time efficient.

To minimize your total downtime between sets, do supersets - utilizing opposing muscle groups in sequence.

For example:

- Go from doing a bicep exercise to a triceps exercise.
- Or work your quadriceps followed by your hamstrings.
- Go from an upper-body exercise to a lower-body exercise.

In this manner, you allow one muscle group to rest while another works, as opposed to sitting idle after doing three chest exercises in order to allow the muscles to recover for the next set.

Also remember to work the large muscle groups before the smaller ones. Chest and back before biceps, triceps and shoulders. Why? When working the larger muscle groups, for example, in the chest press, the smaller muscles of the arms assist. If they are already fatigued, they won't ensure the safety of the exercise or allow you the proper support you need to lift the heavier weights.

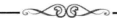

Circuit training allows you to burn more calories by working a greater number of muscles in less time.

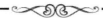

Lauren's Love: My Favourite Circuit Workout

It involves 10 exercises of 50 reps each (700 reps total). It's efficient, generally requiring only 25–30 minutes; elevates my heart rate, and definitely keeps me toned and maintains my muscle mass.

I change the exercises in my circuit at least every month in order to prevent my body from getting used to the workout and my mind from getting bored. Or, I will alternate between different circuit workouts within the same week.

Here is my current **700 Rep Total Conditioning Circuit Workout**; it targets all the major muscle groups. Go to **www.change4good.ca** to both download and see demonstrations of all these exercises.

1. Step-ups using a bench (50 reps on each leg)
2. Push-ups using a Bosu, if available (50 reps)
3. Seated rows using a resistance band (50 reps)
4. Full crunches with a dumbbell (50 reps) and seated dumbbell oblique twists (20 reps)
5. Glute dips using a stability ball (50 reps on each leg)
6. Tricep dips using a stability ball (50 reps)
7. Biceps curls using a resistance band or dumbbells (50 reps)
8. Squat jumps (50 reps)
9. V-sits with/without a dumbbell (30 reps) and leg toss with/without a stability ball (20 reps)
10. Walking lunges (50 reps on each leg)

I either start or finish the workout by doing 6 different plank exercises to give my core muscles that extra boost.

As you can see you also do not need expensive equipment to be able to do an effective workout at home (or when you travel). However, for those who insist, here are some of my favourite 'toys':

1. **Incline-decline bench or step with risers.**
2. **Free weights** – dumbbells.
3. **Stability ball** – allows you to train the entire body and is especially good for the core. The instability of the ball forces the use of stabilizing muscles. To select the proper size: thighs should be parallel to the ground when sitting.
4. **Resistance tubing** – provides a variety of levels of resistance; portable.
5. **TRX Suspension Trainers** - a system that uses your own body weight to create resistance.
6. **Medicine ball** (weighted rubber ball) – with or without handles.
7. **Skipping rope.**
8. **Bosu** - a half-sphere on a flat platform - great for improving balance.
9. **Body Bar.**
10. **Foam Roller.**
11. **Mini trampoline.**
12. **Mini hurdles.**

5. **Eccentric Training**

   Eccentric training refers to the lowering phase of an exercise. The slower this eccentric or lowering phase the larger the challenge to the muscle. Eccentric exercise translates into a longer rebuilding process and a greater post-workout metabolic increase.

It takes gravity and momentum out of the equation. You control the weight as it reaches the bottom, and then pause for a moment before lifting again. Essentially, you work as hard and in as controlled a manner whether you are lifting or lowering a weight.

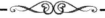

Eccentric exercise translates into a longer rebuilding process and a greater post-workout metabolic increase.

6. Weight Training or Cardio First?

The second most common question I am asked is whether to do weight training or cardiovascular training first. The answer depends on your primary workout goal. Is it to improve body composition? Is it to improve your cardiovascular endurance? Or is your goal to improve your muscular strength?

- **If your primary focus is to improve body composition** – which means burn fat and improve the ratio of lean tissue to fat (we obviously want more lean tissue and less fat) – then **do weight/strength training first** (after a warm-up).

  Why? For most of us, effective fat burning begins approximately 20 minutes into our workout routine. (It begins sooner if you are more fit because well-conditioned muscles utilize fat as a preferred source of energy sooner than untrained muscles).

  By doing weight training first, you are invoking a stress response that frees up fatty acids while you are getting the benefits of a strength workout.

Once you begin your cardio routine, those fatty acids are available to be burned through the cardio activity, right from the start, which is the primary goal of a cardio workout, besides of course improving cardiovascular fitness.

- Similarly, **if your primary goal is to develop muscular strength, do your strength workout before your cardio workout.**

  Muscles rested, you'll have optimal energy to lift heavier weights. If you do your cardio workout first, your muscles will be somewhat fatigued.

  Doing your cardio workout immediately after the strength workout can also speed up recovery by supplying the muscles with more oxygen and removing muscular waste products accumulated during strength training.

  Keeping the cardio workout at a low to moderate intensity will keep the muscles from getting too sore after your workout. It will also improve your cardiovascular and respiratory fitness (lung power), while assisting muscle recovery.

- **If your primary focus**, however, is **developing cardiovascular endurance**, being able to do a longer, sustained cardio workout (30-60+ minutes), then **do your cardio first** while your muscles are fresh.

A note about energy: The higher the intensity of the workout, the more sugar your body uses as fuel. When working at a lower intensity, you tend to use more fat.

However, you are always burning a proportion of both fat and sugar. The most important goal for weight reduction or weight maintenance is to work at as high intensity as possible in order to **burn as many calories as possible.** Although the percentage of fat burnt may be slightly lower, the overall number of calories and amount of fat burnt will be greater which is, after all, the goal when you're trying to lose weight and increase muscle to fat ratio. **Remember, regardless of what you do first, warm-up and cool down afterwards.**

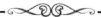

The most important goal for weight reduction or weight maintenance is to work at as high intensity as possible in order to burn as many calories as possible.

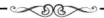

6. Train in the Morning or Later in the Day?

Another popular question: better to work out first thing in the morning or later in the day? Both have advantages.

- First, it's best to work out when you have the time, which could even be midday, and when you have the most energy. Exercising in the morning allows us to benefit from the body's higher metabolic rate through the rest of the day. No matter what you do after your exercise session, your body will be burning more calories for the next few hours.

- However exercising later in the day helps stimulate our metabolism, which naturally starts to slow down as the day wanes.

- For these reasons, either is good. Personally, I prefer mornings. Later in the day, I struggle to do a good workout as *my* energy level isn't as high. I try to schedule time for my workouts as early in my day as possible. In that fashion, it done no matter what later surprises the day brings.

7. Technique

Technique, technique, technique – especially when it comes to lifting weights, technique is everything. Make sure your body positions are correct for all exercises.

In this regard, a good trainer is vital. If you don't have access to one, read books on fitness (in addition to this one) and study pictures and videos. The slightest misalignment can mean possible injury or failure to work the intended muscle group properly.

If nothing else, remember:

- Perform slow, controlled reps, both when you lift and lower the weight.

- Maintain a strong core contraction during all exercises whether you are standing, sitting or lying down.

- Finally, visually focus on the muscle group you are working. This ensures that you are targeting the intended muscles, and will reduce the risk of injury. In addition, the visualization in this context has been shown to recruit muscle fibres to a greater extent.

8. Plyometrics

Plyometrics is a fancy word for hop, skip and jump. Essentially, it's **an advanced strength training technique that emphasizes bounding and explosive movements.** It places increased stress on the joints and connective tissue – and has a higher risk of injury – but it also helps increase the fitness and strength gained through an exercise. An example of a plyometric exercise is jumping on and off a platform or squat jumps. Beginners should avoid plyometrics.

9. Avoid overtraining

When you exercise for too long within one session (typically more than 2 hours), your body senses stress. Cortisol is released, and as you know, cortisol increases appetite and fat storage.

Chronic over-training also leads to:
- Decreased performance and fitness gains.
- Compromised recovery.
- A suppressed immune system.
- An elevated resting heart rate.
- Possibly even depression.

Remember, quality is more important than quantity. Take a day or two of rest each week. On your rest days, do recreational activities that are not what you typically do – hike, play golf. Anything less intense and varied will do the trick.

From Theory to Practice

As we learned in earlier chapters, motivation is the issue. Can you be consistent? Can you hang in for the long haul? Can you make fitness a pleasurable part of daily life? **Here are a dozen tips to show you how:**

1. **Have a schedule.** Know which days of the week and what time you are going to work out. If you do not schedule your workouts each week, life will intervene and before you know it, the week will be gone and your fitness journal will be blank (see page 344).I schedule all my workouts in my BlackBerry™ through the next year – literally. If for some reason I can't make a scheduled workout, I won't book the new appointment unless I can reschedule the workout. **Discipline keeps you on track.**

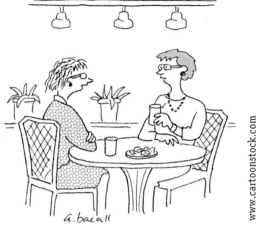

"I started a serious workout program yesterday. So far I missed only one session."

www.cartoonstock.com

a.bacall

2. **Set sustainable REAL SMART GOALS** (see Chapter TWO). Don't leap from the couch into a 5km race during your first workout. Start slowly and gradually build duration and intensity. This way, you'll prevent injury, feel accomplished and remain motivated. Also, a qualified and experienced personal trainer can help.

3. **Monitor your progress in an exercise journal.**

   You can download the Change4Good Exercise Journal© at **www.change4good.ca**, (see a sample on the next page). Just like you write down what you eat, keep track of your workouts.

   See your progress and where and when you need to change your routine. Monitor your intensity within your workout. Use a heart rate monitor or any other method to make sure you're actually improving. You could monitor the calories you burn per session, or the distance you cover – any objective measure will do. Then – write it down.

Sample Change4Good Exercise Journal

Change4Good Exercise Journal©   Date: *July 18 – 24 2011*

My commitment to exercising is:

Cardio: _____3 - 4_____ times per week for _____30 - 45_____ minutes per session

Weights: _____2 - 3_____ times per week for _____30 - 45_____ minutes per session

I will work out on the following days: Ⓜ Ⓣ Ⓦ T Ⓕ Ⓢ Ⓢ

Strength Training	Date			Date			Date			Date			Date			Date			Date		
Muscle Group:				*July 19*						*July 21*												
Chest	W	S	R	W	S	R	W	S	R	W	S	R	W	S	R	W	S	R	W	S	R
Push up - Wide				BW	1	30				BW	1	30									
DB - Fly				25	1	15				25	1	15									
Push Up - Decline				BW	1	20				BW	1	20									
Back	W	S	R	W	S	R	W	S	R	W	S	R	W	S	R	W	S	R	W	S	R
Wide Pulldown				8P	1	15				8P	1	15									
Reverse Fly (DB)				10	1	15				10	1	15									
Seated Row				8P	1	15				8P	1	15									
Triceps	W	S	R	W	S	R	W	S	R	W	S	R	W	S	R	W	S	R	W	S	R
Kickbacks (DB)				12	2	15				12	2	15									
Dips (SB)				BW	2	20				BW	2	20									
Biceps	W	S	R	W	S	R	W	S	R	W	S	R	W	S	R	W	S	R	W	S	R
Hammer Curl (DB)				15	1	15				15	1	15									
Concentration Curl				20	1	15				20	1	15									
Shoulders	W	S	R	W	S	R	W	S	R	W	S	R	W	S	R	W	S	R	W	S	R
Side Raises (DB)				8	1	15				8	1	15									
Legs	W	S	R	W	S	R	W	S	R	W	S	R	W	S	R	W	S	R	W	S	R
Bench Step Ups				15	1	15				15	1	15									
Lying Leg Curl				3P	1	15				3P	1	15									
Regular Squats				35	1	15				35	1	15									
Hamstring Pull In				SB	1	20				SB	1	20									
Walking Lunges				20	1	15				20	1	15									
Abs/Core	W	S	R	W	S	R	W	S	R	W	S	R	W	S	R	W	S	R	W	S	R
Full Crunch (DB)				30	2	30				30	2	30									
Seated Twist (DB)				20	1	30				20	1	30									
Leg Toss (SB)				SB	1	20				SB	1	20									

Cardio Workout	Date	Date	Date	Date	Date	Date	Date
	July 18	*July 19*	*July 20*	*July 21*	*July 22*		*July 24*
Exercise	Elliptical	Weights	Run	Weights	Elliptical		Walk
Time	45 min	45 min	30 min	45 min	45 min		90 min
Distance	8 km		5 km		8 km		11-12 km
Intensity/HR	75 – 80%	8/10 RPE	75 – 80%	8/10 RPE	75 – 80%		75 – 90%
Calories Burned	580		350		575		600

Legend: DB = Dumbbells | BW = Body Weight | P = Plates | SB = Stability Ball | RB = Resistance

Change4Good Exercise Journal©

Change4Good Exercise Journal©   Date:

My commitment to exercising is:

Cardio: _____ times per week for _____ minutes per session

Weights: _____ times per week for _____ minutes per session

I will work out on the following days: M   T   W   T   F   S   S

Strength Training	Date			Date			Date			Date			Date			Date			Date		
Muscle Group:																					
Chest	W	S	R	W	S	R	W	S	R	W	S	R	W	S	R	W	S	R	W	S	R
Back	W	S	R	W	S	R	W	S	R	W	S	R	W	S	R	W	S	R	W	S	R
Triceps	W	S	R	W	S	R	W	S	R	W	S	R	W	S	R	W	S	R	W	S	R
Biceps	W	S	R	W	S	R	W	S	R	W	S	R	W	S	R	W	S	R	W	S	R
Shoulders	W	S	R	W	S	R	W	S	R	W	S	R	W	S	R	W	S	R	W	S	R
Legs	W	S	R	W	S	R	W	S	R	W	S	R	W	S	R	W	S	R	W	S	R
Abs/Core	W	S	R	W	S	R	W	S	R	W	S	R	W	S	R	W	S	R	W	S	R

Cardio Workout	Date	Date	Date	Date	Date	Date	Date
Exercise							
Time							
Distance							
Intensity/HR							
Calories Burned							

Legend: DB = Dumbbells | BW = Body Weight | P = Plates | SB = Stability Ball | RB = Resistance

Move: Exercise at Least 30-60 Minutes Every Day

4. **Plan not only when you will work out but exactly what you will do – and stick to it.** I always know exactly what I will do when I walk into the gym. Some days I finish my weight training in 35 minutes; other days I do it in 25 minutes, but regardless, I finish the entire routine.

5. **Workout with a friend.** Having a training buddy makes workouts more fun and you more accountable. Your workout buddy should be as motivated – or preferably more motivated than you are.

6. **Music is a great mood changer and energy up-lifter.** I never do cardio without my iPod.

7. **Hire a trainer** if you are new to training or if you need a change in workout. A qualified, experienced trainer will make sure you exercise with proper form, and that you are doing exercises necessary to meet your goals. Also, paying ensures that you'll show up.

8. **Join a team.** If you enjoy group sports or activities, join a soccer team or baseball league. Join a running group. It will provide support, new friends and nudge you to stay committed.

9. **Sign up for an event.** Fun run/walks for charity are always good options. They give you focus and a goal.

10. **Buy a pedometer.** It's a great, inexpensive tool for beginners that will help you track the number of steps you take per day. Using it allows you to measure your progress precisely. Aim for 10,000 steps daily. Soon, you'll find out how addictive it can be. Involve the family in a contest or challenge your office buddies.

11. **Make sure you have clothes that are comfortable, and appropriate** for both the activity you are doing and the weather. Also, walking around in cool exercise gear is enormously motivating. Pay special attention to shoes. Make sure yours are suited to the activity and not old or worn out. Remember, shoes aren't meant to last forever....neither is your body so use it well and wisely. The payoff is tremendous.

12. **Have Fun.**

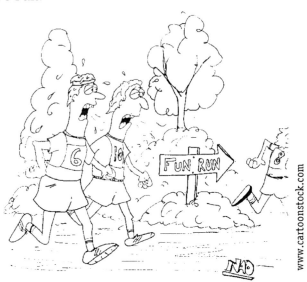

"Are we having fun yet?!"

CHANGE4GOOD – ACTION STEPS

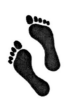

- Start implementing Principle 10 – Move: Exercise at least 30–60 minutes every day (aiming for 5 hrs. a week).
- Complete your Change4Good Fitness GPS©.
- Create and implement your exercise plan (hire a trainer if necessary).
- Identify and complete your ninth short-term (weekly) goal. For example: join a running group; buy a pedometer; block off time each day to workout and/or register for a charity fun run.
- Update Change4Good Journal© daily.
- Update Change4Good Goal Sheet© weekly.
- Start and then update daily your Change4Good Exercise Journal©.

TOOLS

- Change4Good Goal Sheet©
- Change4Good Journal©
- Change4Good Fitness GPS©
- Lauren's 700Rep Circuit Total Conditioning Workout©
- Change4Good Exercise Journal©

REMEMBER THIS

- From the laws of physics – it's easier to keep a body in motion than to get it in motion. The moral of the story; KEEP MOVING.

CONCLUSION

In this book, and now I hope in your head, is the bedrock, I believe, of what you need to know – and do – to remain fit, healthy and I hope, happy in terms of nutrition and exercise. It is also my belief that the overall sanity with which I've tried to imbue the Change4Good program will seep into other areas of your life as well. Feeling good, looking good and being good – well, in some ways they're all connected.

As a formerly chronic dieter, I fully understand the excitement that attends the start of any kind of sweeping change one undertakes to improve his/her life. Let's first of all, get a little better understanding of that word sweeping. If you follow the Change4Good principles in their entirety, and you follow them consistently – you will achieve an incredible change in your life. It just won't happen overnight. And that's good news, because overnight changes tend to vanish by the morning. They will be sweeping, however, in the sense that they will carry you along – people tend to do what they see working – and they will encompass every area of your life. To me this sounds like an awful lot to receive for merely following ten very simple directives.

Of course as I've shared many times, simple doesn't mean easy. Anyone can drink 8 glasses of water a day – but will you? That's the question. Habits, even small ones, are hard to establish. In the beginning, even the smallest, simplest changes require attention, focus and commitment. If towards the end of Day 3 you see you've only drunk 4 glasses of water, do you have the energy to run back into the house and grab your water bottle? And will you do it each time you forget it? A habit, however hard to establish, eventually becomes easy to sustain.

I focus on this tiny change – Principle 9 – because it's such an easy one and yet it illustrates the larger point: discipline is contagious. Once you actually do put in the (mental and physical) effort to follow even one of these principles consistently, how beautifully you'll see the others falling into place. As if by magic, you'll suddenly find yourself saying no to the gang who always corrals you into drinking more than you want to every Friday night and turning instead to the friend who wants to go for a run along the river.

Our bodies want us to be healthy; they're made that way. If you treat them right, they'll surprise you by leading you, almost without much effort on your part, to the gorgeous bowl of fruit on the counter rather than to the wilting soggy pie. I'm no stranger to dessert, as you know; even at my currently healthy goal weight, you can find me almost every weekend digging into a favorite treat, but as you know from the chapter on eating out, I've "earned" the right to that lovely piece of cheese cake – I've exercised 30-60 minutes every day and I've practiced Principle 8 (moderation). I'm not ordering the nachos or the beer; I'm giving them up for the cheesecake. That way, when I do weigh myself, even the scale won't seem to register the fact that I've actually eaten my favorite food. In short, weight that seemed impossible to get off initially now stays off with remarkable ease. Instead of bellyaching about all that you do have to give up (and you might in the beginning), suddenly you're exclaiming – I can't believe how much and how well I get to eat and still I'm the right weight – plus, I can run a half marathon in a shorter time or my flab is gone or (substitute in your particular goal).

The deal is: you put the effort in up front and all that determination and consistency will reward you with what appears to be an effort-less healthy lifestyle in the end. It worked for me; it works for hundreds of my clients, it will work for you. Just do your part (and if you've forgotten what it is, go back to Chapter ONE) and a happier healthier you will be your reward.

A few final reminders:

1. Don't cut corners. In the beginning, go ahead. Be obsessive. Spend hours, even days if you insist, laboring over your goals and food and exercise journals and make sure everything is intact. Pick a time in your life when you have a little extra free mental energy to apply it to Change4Good. Then, when the deluge from work or from family problems starts to hit – and it always will – you'll have enough experience under your belt so that a more healthy way of living and being will come to you second nature.

2. Have faith. If that scale doesn't budge the first week, go back and honestly see what you're possibly doing wrong. Which principle did you skimp on? If you're having trouble with any of them, see what in your life can change to accommodate them. Keep your eyes on the goal – never question it – and you'll have the energy to overcome obstacles as they arise. And not only will you turn into a thinner, fitter person, you'll turn into an emotionally stronger one as well.

3. Share it. The best way to keep something wonderful is to give it away. Ask a few friends to join you. Have weekly meetings or email fetes in which you can all monitor each other's goals every week, commiserate, share tips, even discuss lifestyle problems. Society is growing more and more isolated; we're all at home alone in front of our computers. Organize Change4Good dinners or walks or simply just water-drinking meetings once a week and give each other support. And don't compete. Share and help and nudge each other along.

4. Finally, and I can't emphasize this strongly enough, let the good sense of these principles seep into the rest of your life. Working too hard? Moderate. Playing too hard? Moderate.

Feeling down and pessimistic and negative about life? Do whatever you can to change reality (go back to your Goal Sheet and Chapter TWO) and if that doesn't work, see what you can do about that old nemesis, a bad attitude. Focusing on solutions instead of problems, expressing gratitude, giving love instead of waiting to receive it – it all helps to make the tough days a little easier to endure.

When first I embarked on the lengthy process that resulted in the Change4Good Program, I was not the happiest human being. No area of my life really satisfied me and it all manifested itself in an unhealthy manner of eating and living. More than a decade later, I have a terrific home, a healthy and fit body, great friends and family members, and a career that I enjoy so much that even on a Saturday – often a busy day with clients -- I can't wait to go into work.

Which is not to say that I don't have tough days – I still "obsess" (it's in my personality) – but the tough days come and then they go. And when I fall, I never fall as hard and I get up so much more quickly. Life is good because I put in the hard work of figuring out how to make it that way. And now, my greatest pleasure has been to share what I've learned with you – all condensed into ten easy principles – simple but not easy; simple, but extremely worthwhile.

A final farewell: As you Change4Good your life, I want to hear about your progress and success. Tell me about your roadblocks as well and problems that keep you from reaching your goals. Use my website and blog as your official hand-holder: on it, post your comments and read those of others. In this way, we'll have a community of Change4Good friends as a source of strength and fellowship. Together, we can all Change4Good – for good.

Sincerely,
Lauren Jawno
www.jawno.com
www.change4good.ca

REFERENCES

PAGE	#	REFERENCE SOURCE
6	1	Quotes by Jim Rohn, America's Foremost Business Philosopher, reprinted with permission from Jim Rohn International ©2011.
6	2	Quotes by Jim Rohn, America's Foremost Business Philosopher, reprinted with permission from Jim Rohn International ©2011.
7	3	Wansink, Brian. Under the Influence: How External Cues Make Us Overeat. Nutrition Action Health Letter: Centre for Science in the Public Interest. May 2011 – Volume 38 – Number 4.
7	4	Wansink, Brian. Under the Influence: How External Cues Make Us Overeat. Nutrition Action Health Letter: Centre for Science in the Public Interest. May 2011 – Volume 38 – Number 4.
42	5	American Council on Exercise. www.acefitness.org
46	6	American Journal of Preventive Medicine. 2008. August: 35(2): 118-126.
102	7	Berardi, John. M. The Precision Nutrition Diet Guide. Science Link Inc (2005)
107	8	http://www.deathtodiabetes.com/uploads/GI-GL_Food_Chart_--_Death_to_Diabetes_-_3pg.pdf
111	9	www.mayoclinic.com/health/artificial-sweeteners/MY00073/NSECTIONGROUP=2
112	10	Colditz GA, Willett WC, Stampfer MJ, London SJ, Segal MR, Speizer FE. Patterns of weight change and their relation to diet in a cohort of healthy women. American Journal of Clinical Nutrition. 1990;'51:1100-1105.
112	11	Stellman SD, Garfinkel L. Artificial sweetner use and one-year weight change among women. Prev. Med. 1986;15:195-202.
117	12	Berardi, John M. The Precision Nutrition Diet Guide, Science Link Inc. (2005).

ABOUT THE AUTHOR

LAUREN JAWNO, the creator and author of the Change4Good Program, has a Bachelors Degree in Education, is a certified nutritionist, fitness trainer, cutting edge wellness and lifestyle coach and media personality. During her 15 years in the field, her clients have included professional corporations including: AB Sciex, Ceridian, Royal Bank of Canada and Mercedes-Benz. Her many private clients include people from all walks of life: doctors, lawyers, business executives, stay-at-home moms, nationally ranked swimmers and runners, hockey and soccer players, world ranked dancers and athletes of all stripes.

A popular member of the respected Health Sciences faculty at Centennial College in Toronto, Lauren is also affiliated with a select group of leading sports and health and wellness facilities in Toronto. A dynamic speaker and frequent guest on television and radio on the subject of fitness, nutrition and lifestyle, Lauren has also written for and been featured in numerous national publications and is a regular columnist for iRun magazine.

Lauren currently resides in Toronto, when not returning to visit family and friends in her native Cape Town, South Africa.

For information on how to contact Lauren Jawno for private consultation, media appearances and public speaking; please go to her website at www.jawno.com.

ABOUT THE CO-AUTHOR

FRAN SCHUMER has 35 years' experience as a reporter, writer, and teacher. She is a best-selling co-author whose stories have appeared on the cover of New York Magazine and in the pages of the New York Times Sunday Magazine, Barron's, Vogue, the Nation and other national publications. She is a graduate of Harvard College and the New York City public schools.

INDEX

P

Percentage Daily Value, 192
Pesco vegetarians, 284
Phospholipids, 122, 126
Phosphorous, 151, 269, 273, 274, 277
Phytic Acid, 277
Phytochemicals, 112
Pilates, 323
Plyometrics, 341
Pollo vegetarians, 284
Polychlorinated biphenyls, 120
Portion control, 7, 133, 176, 207, 211,
   215, 243
Price Look Up number, 283
Principle 1, xxxiii, 1, 18, 24, 60, 200, 210
Principle 10, xxxvii, 299, 348
Principle 2, xxiii, xxxiv, 27, 57, 230, 327
Principle 3, xxxiv, 59, 88
Principle 4, xxxiv, 60, 91, 95, 133, 138,
   265, 302, 305
Principle 5, xxxv, 60, 79, 82, 104, 141,
   142, 170, 173, 179, 181, 203
Principle 7, xxxvi, 60, 205, 225, 306
Principle 8, xxxi, xxxvi, 60, 78, 212, 227,
   245, 350
Principle 9, xxxvii, 247, 295, 350
Probiotics, 273, 294
Progressive Overload, 327
Protein, xxxiv, 44, 50, 79, 80, 81, 91, 92,
   93, 95, 96, 98, 99, 100, 103, 108, 115,
   116, 117, 118, 119, 120, 121, 128,
   131, 132, 138, 143, 146, 154, 170,
   171, 172, 174, 176, 188, 193, 207,
   208, 209, 215, 220, 224, 225, 229,
   232, 240, 244, 248, 259, 266, 270,
   274,276, 285, 288, 289, 292, 294, 301,
   302, 303, 306, 307
   Protein powder, 50

Q

Quadriceps, 318

R

Quinoa, 98, 113, 115, 119, 136, 138, 174,
   232, 259, 260, 285

R

Range of motion, 314, 324
Rating of Perceived Exertion, 320
Repetitions, 321, 326, 334
Resistance bands, 313, 323, 336
Restaurants, 209, 228, 229, 233, 234,
   235, 241, 242
Reverse osmosis, 168
Reversibility, 329
Riboflavin, 145, 194

S

Sacha inchi seeds, 138
Seeds, 103, 115, 124, 125, 127, 133, 161,
   179, 202, 209, 219, 223, 230, 275,
   277, 285, 286, 289, 295
Semi vegetarians, 284
Serving size, 183, 184
Shoulders, 318
Skin, xxx, xxxv, 41, 125, 129, 146, 162,
   164, 253, 254, 261, 262, 278, 280, 293
Skin Brushing, 262
Skipping rope, 337
Sleep, 15, 65, 69, 70, 71, 72, 73, 86, 290,
   311
Soy, 114, 115, 119, 222, 274, 285
Specificity of Training, 326
Spirulina, 115, 260, 285
Split program, 318
Stability ball, 336
Stanols, 122, 127
Starch, 185, 186, 187
Steroid Hormones, 129
Strength training, 119, 307, 313, 314,
   321, 323, 331, 333, 334, 338, 339, 341
Stress, 308
Super Foods, 291, 292, 293, 294
Supersized, 216

CPSIA information can be obtained at www.ICGtesting.com
Printed in the USA
LVOW080614080213

319159LV00003B/11/P